Listening
to the
Animals

NOEL FITZPATRICK

Becoming The Supervet

Listening to the Animals

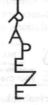

An Orion Paperback

First published in Great Britain in 2018
by Trapeze
This paperback edition published in 2019
By Trapeze, an imprint of The Orion Group Ltd,
Carmelite House, 50 Victoria Embankment,
London EC4Y 0DZ

An Hachette UK company

1 3 5 7 9 10 8 6 4 2

A CIP catalogue record for this book is available
from the British Library.

ISBN (Paperback): 978 1 409 18376 1

Typeset by Input Data Services Ltd, Somerset

Printed and bound in Great Britain by Clays Ltd, Elcograf S.p.A.

The Orion Publishing Group's policy is to use papers that
are natural, renewable and recyclable products and
made from wood grown in sustainable forests. The logging
and manufacturing processes are expected to conform to
the environmental regulations of the country of origin.

*To all of the animals and humans
who have inspired me, loved me
and been my friends.*

CONTENTS

CHAPTER ONE

The Lamb

The Birth of The Supervet

The mackerel stripes of a brightly freezing moon grabbed at the clouds and crept through my ice-scribbled bedroom window. My small white rickety bed had a very thin mattress on even thinner springs that squeaked with every movement, so I tried my best to remain still. My bedroom was one of five in an old stone farmhouse, and, being furthest from the chimney breast, was so cold that you could write your name on the frosted windowpane. If your leg fell out of bed in the middle of the night, when you woke up you'd think that someone had chopped it off. It was still warmer than outside, though. A family of mice had set up house behind the skirting board and had gnawed a big hole in the flowery wallpaper. Mammy had put out the mousetrap but because I couldn't bear to wake up and find one dead in it, I kept covering it up with a T-shirt.

I wasn't long in bed, it seemed, when the alarm went off. It was a big old green-and-white metal alarm clock with a tick-tock that I hated, and I still hate that noise to this day. Another trusty T-shirt was used to muffle the sound, but this

1

didn't stop the ferocious clang of the two bells and the little hammer at the top of it. It was time to get up and check on the sheep. It was 1978 and I was ten years old. During lambing season throughout spring, Daddy always did the morning shift and I always did the night shift at one or two o'clock in the morning, which probably goes some way to explain why I'm a night owl. One thing is for sure: I am not a morning person.

In 1970s Ballyfin, in County Laois in the Republic of Ireland, lambing was generally an outdoors pursuit. Well, it certainly was on the farm of Sean Fitzpatrick, my father. There wasn't enough shed space to house the ewes before they lambed. Only once they had lambed or if you thought they were going to have a lamb imminently could they be brought in out of the cold. Of course, this was frequently misjudged, and they lambed in the field.

I plunged from the snug, squeaky bed into the cold darkness, the wisps of moonlight like freezing icicles jabbing my feet. It was so cold I layered up quickly, pulling an old jumper over my checked pyjamas, then my padded green jacket, a woolly hood over my tousled mop of hair, and trousers that were too big for me by virtue of being handed down from my older brother. I often had an image of being frozen to the spot like someone petrified by very cold lava from a frozen volcano. Stumbling through the yellow door of my bedroom, which to this day is still adorned with a very small china plaque saying 'Private', I knocked two of the key rings I collected off the nails on the wall, one a small soldier. That's what I felt like: a small lambing soldier. Downstairs by the door of our back kitchen, I pulled oversized wellies onto my skinny little legs and marched out into the black night.

February frost had starched the fields in silent rigidity, and only the muffled bleating of sheep in various states of restless awakening and the quiet sounds of lambs slipping on the grass or eagerly nuzzling the udders of their mothers were palpable through the half-moonlight. I did the head-count: fifty-seven. Where was number fifty-eight? Fecking hell, I'd have to tour the ditches. Being surrounded by deep drains along the hedgerows, the fields at home were woefully equipped to deal with lambing, but that was just the way it was. It wasn't until much later that most of the lambing was done in a shed bedded with straw. Oh, the luxury!

About twenty minutes into my sub-arctic trek I found her, half-drowned at the bottom of one of the deep drainage ditches, struggling to keep her head above the freezing surface, half-dead with exhaustion yet half-alive in the throes of labour. Even at that age, I had a couple of years' experience of lambing sheep, and my wee hands worked in my favour. There was no way that I was going to be able to haul the ewe up the sloping bank and out of the ditch which was about four or five feet deep, so I slid down on the frosty mud alongside her. Her rear end was submerged so I rolled up my sleeve and delved through the freezing water, putting my small hand into the ewe's birth canal. It was the weirdest combination of biting cold and kind-of-warm moist birth passage. The lamb was stuck, head down in front of the pelvic inlet with one leg facing my hand. *Shit. Bollocks*. In doing so much forbidden cursing in my head, at least I wouldn't have to sin by inventing non-existent sins in next Friday's confessional: I'd actually have something to confess!

I was not good at many things at that age; in fact, I'd say I was good at absolutely nothing at all, except lambing sheep. I pushed on the lamb's head until it was back further into the womb, which wasn't that hard because by now the mother was hardly pushing at all. Then I pushed the leading leg in after it beyond the pelvis. That is the trick; you'd never get the other front leg up and into the pelvis and the birth canal unless you got the leading leg and the head back in first. Then my small hand ran from the one leg to the other over the breast bone until two little claweens popped up – upsy-daisy, there we go, get the nose up between the front legs, steady the head between the knuckles of the front feet, keep both legs moving out of the birth canal by holding onto the knuckles, with a second hand holding the skull in place by the eye sockets – and pull, baby, pull. And I did, with such ferocity that I was flung back on my arse into the sub-zero ditchwater with a tiny female lamb on my chest.

I clawed back up the bank, a damp slimy urchin, and tried to pump the lamb's chest. I swung the little girl back and forth by the back legs, slapping the chest on each swing. I'd done this many times before and had seen Daddy do it for as long as I could remember. I got some reeds and poked the nostrils trying to evoke a snort. I put my mouth down over her nose and I sucked out the mucus and spat it on the grass. I sucked and I blew, I poked reeds and I slapped that little chest but nary a splutter. She was dead. '*Bollocks*.' Now I had at least two sins for First Friday mass night, plus I was an abject failure. '*Damn. Bollocks.*'

I kneeled there on the grass, looking at the dead lamb on one side and the gasping ewe on the other, lying still on the slippery bank of the ditch, knackered. The expectation of impending admonishment from Daddy resonated like thunder in my head. It was definitely my fault. All my fault. I momentarily pulled myself together and tried to encourage the poor ewe out of the ditch. She was exhausted and having

4

none of it. As I pulled on her head and her front legs, she moved not an inch. So I had to slide back down the slimy ditch bank a second time. I tried to push her rear to encourage her to clamber out, and it was as if she was pushing against me. Pushing against me, that was it! Damn, there could be another one in there! I put my hand into the birth passage again and there he or she was, arse first, tail hanging out. I'd have to perform a complete rotation under the icy water or deliver it breach.

I pushed the lamb's backside back in and both back legs immediately popped up. Right, breach it is then! I pulled like mad and out came a male lamb in one smooth tug. Up we launched onto the bank, and this time I would not be beaten. Same thing all over again – pummelling, swinging, prodding, sucking, blowing. A gasp, a splutter. Yes! Alive! *C'mon baby, c'mon baby lamb, let's go, let's go.* A few more swings and there he was – at least a few breaths. Better still, the ewe was struggling to get out of the drain. I slid back down a third time and gave her a push and up she clambered, with the drive only a mother wanting desperately to lick her newborn lamb could have. And so she did. But it was freezing there, absolutely brass-knacker freezing, so I scooped up the lamb and trudged on back towards the relative comfort of a shed near our house. 'C'mon Mrs, C'mon Mrs! *Gin, gin gin gin . . .* C'mon.' By the way, I don't know to this day why throughout my entire youth we called sheep with the phrase 'gin gin'. I guess it's some kind of ancient sheep language handed down through the shepherding ages.

I was about halfway back up the field when my feet failed me. I slipped on the grass and my little lamb was flung out in front of me, with the mother frantically nuzzling him. I was no more than a foot away from him when one last small, warm sigh blurred into my foggy eyes and he breathed his last. *No, no, no, no, no, no! Please, God, no*, I screamed inside.

The lamb was dead. The mum looked up at me with big confused eyes. She looked back at the lamb and tried forlornly to lick a breath back into him. I was trembling with helplessness, abject desolation and dread, hunched down and rocking back and forth holding my knees as I watched her desperately trying to lick the life back into the slimy, limp little body, growing colder by the second.

I rolled over on my back. The fog-frosted dew closed around me on the grass, the ice-cold air ripping my thumping heart out of my chest. I looked up at all the stars in the firmament, tears streaming from my eyes and freezing on my cheeks as they fell. I just stared up at the enormity of it all, still, utterly alone and wretched, and the big yellow moon stared back down at me. The entire universe was witness to my pitiful, utter uselessness. I remember it vividly as if it were yesterday, and I have remembered it many times since – screaming at the sky, one long guttural anguished cry. The poor sheep lay down beside me and gave up too. I found the brightest star in heaven and wished on it with all of my heart that I might be strong enough, brave enough, clever enough, skilled enough and powerful enough. I was none of these things. I felt totally worthless and pathetic.

As it turned out I would feel this way many times in the future when I had tried my best and still lost a life. I'd spend the rest of my life trying not to be useless, trying to save animals, trying against all of the odds to cheat death and keep light in the world, trying to be better than I feel I can ever be, trying to be better than I dream that I could ever be. I have never made it. I still feel like I am never good enough, strong enough, clever enough.

In my work as a veterinary surgeon, I try to inspire light in others – vets that I mentor, kids that I try to influence for good, cynical and jaded people who lie down and give up. I try to get them to listen to the animals – and listen to each other. I believe we are all stars in the firmament and, in my heart of hearts, I am ten years of age forever, wishing that one day, maybe if everyone tried to shine a little light, then the world might be a better place – for us and for all of the animals.

I got the exhausted mother, now without any lambs, back to the safety of the straw shed and trudged back to bed. I crept upstairs hoping not to wake Daddy: I'd leave the explanation for the next day. Rustling around till I found some dry socks and another jumper, I climbed back into bed and huddled under the covers, rubbing my feet to pull some blood back into them after the cold of the drain. My breath painting small clouds of mist on the silent air, I had a sense of the enormity of the challenge ahead crush down upon me like some giant hand of God, so I could barely breathe. Not just the challenge of what I was going to tell Daddy tomorrow, but also the challenge that would face all of my tomorrows. I never wanted to feel that worthless again. I desperately wanted to be strong and clever.

I couldn't sleep. In that lonely blackness I reached for my companion of the night-time; an old Sony transistor radio scavenged some months earlier from a scrap heap and for which I had made an aerial from a coat hanger. I turned it on and lay in the dark with the radio to my ear and started to tune it. I was looking for anything to distract me from the helpless solitude. Hiss, crackle, pop and hiss again, as I slowly turned the black plastic dial. Then all of a sudden the dark bedroom was bathed in the auditory glow of Led Zeppelin's 'Stairway to Heaven'. I'd chanced upon Radio

Luxembourg, the now-defunct pirate radio station. I'd never heard anything like it before or since, and the ethereal song exploded in my mind with infinite possibility. I finally fell asleep building my very own stairway to the stars.

Thank you the Lamb With No Name for allowing me a glimpse of the brightest star in heaven: in listening to you I might one day realise my place among it all. The lamb unsurprisingly did not have a name, but undoubtedly has given me mine. On that fateful night that defined the course of my entire life, you taught me to have humility as well as the highest possible aspirations.

CHAPTER TWO

Cattle, Sheep and Soil

My Daddy, Sean Fitzpatrick

I gulped in my first mouthful of air at about 7 p.m., on Wednesday, 13 December 1967. My Daddy Sean had dropped Mammy Rita off at Laois County Hospital, in Portlaoise, on the previous evening, and then went back to the farm to look after the sheep and the cattle. It was a long and troublesome labour and, because there were no beds available, Mammy was on a gurney in the corridor, from the time of drop-off on the Tuesday, until late the following afternoon, when she was finally taken into the delivery ward. The doctor apparently passed by a few times, tapping her on the belly and saying, 'Bumpety bump, not ready yet, Rita.' She told me that she asked several passers-by for painkillers with the plaintive cry of 'Help me!' – to no avail, of course. Neither physical nor pharmaceutical help was forthcoming. Mammy says that's just how things were done back then. I'm pretty sure that she would have got quicker assistance at my own veterinary practice today!

Daddy wasn't at the birth; it wasn't common practice for fathers to be in the delivery ward, and he was busy working anyway. He came in to see us a couple of hours later, apparently very pleased that he had another boy, and then went back to work. Mammy was in the hospital with me for about a week and a neighbour from a house nearby, Mrs Dunne, who would later become my godmother, looked after my older brother and three sisters. When Mammy was ready to take me home, Daddy didn't have time to come and pick us up because he was busy cutting the horns off cattle. In Daddy's head that was fair enough. I was already in the world, and collecting us was less of a priority than dealing with the cows – the cattle, the sheep and the land came first. Such it was for my father, as it was for his own father, and his father before that.

Daddy was doing the dehorning for Brother Germanus from the Patrician Brothers, the local boys' school, which, twelve years later, I would attend. So, Daddy got on with the job and asked Brother Germanus to fetch us from the hospital. Needless to say, there was many a raised eyebrow among the nurses when 'a man of the collar' entered in his slippers, all smiles, and lifted me up like I was in fact his own, and carried me all bouncy and chattery out of the hospital doors, followed closely by a rather dishevelled, exhausted and entirely blameless Rita. That provided enough gossip for a day or two, no doubt.

I readily admit that I'm very much my father's son in looks and work ethic – and because I grew up working beside him on the farm, I understand why he thought that dehorning cattle was the greater priority. I imagine he probably had run into some bother with the cattle and felt that it was a job that only he could sort out. No doubt he concluded that arranging for an able-bodied, reliable man to collect us was totally justifiable. Let's face it: anyone who could drive a car could do that, whereas in my dad's reasoning, only he could handle the dehorning. I understand that, and have been guilty myself of a similar inability to delegate where animals are involved, but I still wish he'd made a bit more of an effort to see that Mammy and I were OK.

On the bright side, as they say, one man's loss is another man's gain, and indeed Brother Germanus relished his self-appointed role as my unofficial godfather. I was his little man and he liked nothing better than to wake me up in the cradle, and make me either smile or cry with his teeth bouncing up and down on his gums. I was breastfed for the week in hospital only, and after that Mammy had to get back to looking after the other children and the house, while Brother Germanus would sit there with me in his arms, happy as the day was long, giving me my bottle. My earliest childhood memory is of Brother Germanus's false teeth chattering up and down with excitement every time he visited the house.

Then there was a bit of a disagreement at my baptism over what I was to be called, because Daddy wanted to call me Martin after his dad, and there was absolutely no way that Mammy was having that. She insisted there were already too many Martins in the family, and persisted in calling me Noel. Daddy wasn't a bit happy, and belligerently went ahead and had Martin Noel Galgani Fitzpatrick recorded on the birth certificate. Mammy was insistent on placing me under the protection of a saint – a common practice in Ireland – and so it was Galgani, after Saint Gemma Galgani. She kept on calling me Noel anyway – as I was her Christmas baby. So Noel I am, and I'm delighted. In truth, Mammy might well have reasoned that calling me Noel didn't matter anyway, because my father was rarely there during my waking hours, except at night, and even then he generally ignored baby crying anyway. Mammy was left to cope with me, my four older siblings, the occasional calf or lamb she was feeding with a bottle in a shed or in the kitchen, along with the various workmen Daddy sent her way to get fed, in addition to all manner of other challenges.

Daddy came from a big family of nine brothers and sisters. They lived in a townland called Brockera, in the parish of Ballyfin, County Laois, about five miles distant from each of the towns Portlaoise, Mountrath and Mountmellick. His father and his grandfather before him were farmers. They mostly grew what they needed to get by. They had potatoes, vegetables and meat, but money was something that was scarce. Daddy milked cows for a local farmer, for half-a-crown each day, which was two shillings and sixpence. When he was in his mid-teens, he finally saved enough to buy a sheep, which died, and then a calf that also died. He applied for a job as the local postman but didn't get it, which was a blow to his self-esteem. He eked out a living by cycling to town with lettuce and onions to sell, and finally bought another sheep that then had lambs, and so he was on his way to becoming a farmer. He went on the road as soon as he could and began to make a living buying and selling cattle and sheep.

My daddy loved sheep and cattle, but most of all, though, my daddy loved 'the deal'. *The deal* was the thing. It pertained to buying a sheep, a cow or even a piece of land. All three were the lifeblood of my father. By the time he was thirty-three years old and had married my mammy – who was twenty-eight – he had established a reputation as a proficient stockman and was a very good cattle dealer. He was probably better at this than at anything else in his life. He went to cattle fairs all around Ireland, always looking for the *sweet deal*. His favourite town for selling cattle was

Mountrath, where he had his own stall on the street outside O'Callaghan's shop, a much-frequented purveyor of food and household provisions. Once established, nobody was allowed to have that spot other than my daddy. It was a prime location as it had the greatest footfall and therefore greatest potential for sales. Hail, rain or shine – well, usually rain – he was there every week on a Wednesday doing the deal.

When buying cattle, Daddy would travel all over Ireland, often finding a sweet deal somewhere on the west coast. He made a point of being early and getting in first before the other dealers arrived. He'd be at the harbour docks when the farmers from the small islands in the west landed off the ferry with their wild cattle; or, to steal a march, he'd travel down along the route to catch the drovers taking the cattle from the peninsulas on the south-west coast to the fair in a market town. His intention, needless to say, was to get the deal done before the cattle ever got to the fair, whether in Listowel, Cahersiveen, Killarney, Castleisland, Kinsale, Macroom, Castletownbere or other similarly exotic places. He gained quite a reputation, and his services in regard to judging the 'best beast' were sought by many a contract dealer or supplier of animals to the meat trade.

In those days, once the deal was done – completed by both parties spitting on their hands and sealing their verbal agreement with a handshake – Daddy put the cattle he bought on a train to Portlaoise. Then he employed the services of a couple of drovers, at the grand fee of three pennies per beast, to walk them to Mountrath where he grazed them in a field he rented. He only walked them back to Ballyfin when he knew he was keeping them for rearing, in other words growing them for meat. If he decided to sell the cattle, then on fair day, he drove them into the street stall in Mountrath.

All of this walking would later be done by us children, when we were old enough to hold a cattle stick. I wasn't born at the time of the fairs, but when they disappeared in the 1960s and were replaced by purpose-built 'cattle marts', I was often roped into stopping gaps in the hedges, or shouting from behind, as cattle were walked on the roads from fields to market.

My dad's buying tactics had, however, a downside. Sometimes he bought cattle as a small herd and, only after getting them home, did he realise that the group included a 'dud'. One time, he bought several yearlings from an islander and later discovered one of them was totally blind – fine when in transit with the herd, but a total nutter back on the farm in Ballyfin! That same blind bullock drove Mammy crazy. Her job was to mind three babies in the house and to keep this berserk animal safely barricaded in a nearby shed with a broken door. She failed miserably. Inevitably it escaped to roam the countryside and Daddy was livid. In my daddy's vocabulary, understanding, patience and tolerance weren't words commonly found in the same sentence as farming and cattle.

On another occasion, Daddy bought a bullock with a really bad wheeze because of a lung infection, but he didn't know because the seller had paid a melodeon player to position himself to play nearby. The melodeon made quite a racket, so, of course, Daddy couldn't hear a thing from the bullock. This wasn't a common event, though, because when it came to cattle and sheep my daddy was usually on the ball.

Along with his love for cattle and sheep, my daddy loved the land. It was as if the soil itself ran through his veins. He was born of the soil and of the animals and he was at one with them. From humble beginnings Daddy bought, during his lifetime, four separate stretches of land, which together became the family farm. All were in Ballyfin. The first was Cappinrush, and it was there that I went home one week after I was born. When I was two years old, he bought Esker, nestled in the foothills of the Slieve Bloom Mountains, and this became the family home throughout my childhood. He bought two further parcels of land, the first a farm and farmhouse close to his Cappinrush holding and the second in Knocknakearn, which was commonly called the Glebe.

I think he loved the Glebe the best, probably because in reclaiming it from bog land he found the greatest challenge and the greatest reward. In addition, I think he found solitude for his soul there. It was an isolated stretch of bog land at the end of a long boreen (lane) and was filled with bird calls and quiet beauty. With its peaty brown clay, its carpet of rushes and moss, its wild orchids and bog cotton, one could get lost there in timeless occupation, and Daddy frequently did. It was land to which he dedicated twenty years of his life, draining and reclaiming the waterlogged earth to grow grass to graze cattle and sheep, and barley and turnips to feed them. He drained it by 'putting down shores' to carry the water away. He ploughed it, tearing up tons of bog oaks – ancient trees that had fallen and submerged and were preserved in the bog – which would peep up above the surface, snaring many the unwary grass-cutting machine. He loved the soil and very much loved the toil.

Daddy and I spent many days late into the evening, just us together, putting down shores in the Glebe. This involved digging, sometimes by hand and sometimes by machine, multiple very long, narrow trenches that fed into a big open trench – the drain. The big drains separated the fields and the narrow trenches were dug in a herringbone fashion, 7 or so feet apart, like tributaries towards a river. In the narrow trenches we laid clay pipes, usually 12 inches long and 4 inches wide – made out of heat-treated clay, before the era of plastic pipes – end to end. We then surrounded the clay pipes with gravel before the trench was filled in. Clearly the objective of the piped channel was to drain water from the marshy bog land.

I think in terms of actual hours, I spent more of my early youth trying to drain the Glebe than doing anything else. There were, of course, many times when I was working with Daddy alongside my siblings, but it was the evenings when it was just the two of us that I treasured the most. I liked being with him in our own oasis of calm, uninterrupted by anyone. It wasn't that he usually said anything much; it was what wasn't said that was more important. Just the thoughts shared and the knowing looks and the *understanding* that we were doing something special together. Not that it felt all that special in the miserable cold and rain. But sometimes it felt meaningful and precious, that together, father and son, we were reclaiming the land and making it habitable for crops and animals with our own bare hands. It was a feeling of oneness in our attachment to the eternity of the soil and also a oneness with nature, I suppose.

When it rained, we'd run for shelter into a broken-down cottage in the middle of the bog land that allegedly was the home of 'Nelly Cuckoo'. Nelly was a mythical woman who supposedly haunted the cottage. It was an eerie little place amid a copse of alder and sally trees and blackthorn and whin bushes, and it had been built on the site of a famine village and cemetery, which existed there in the late 1840s.

As we were digging up the ground to lay drainage pipes, we unearthed many bones and clay utensils from years gone by. It was said that Nelly had lost her children to the famine and stayed on to look for them. I don't particularly believe in ghosts, but I was always scared in that derelict cottage. One evening, as I was approaching, a strange shadow hung over the bottom half of the door. Apparently, there used to be a half-door at this house, as was common in Irish cottages. It opened like a stable door, with the bottom closed when necessary to keep children inside and animals out. The top half was generally opened to aerate the house (because the windows were so small since glass was expensive), or just to lean on and talk to friends or neighbours. It was this outline of an old woman's shadow on an absent half-door that I encountered. In the warmth of that summer evening there was a chill about the scene. It was probably just a trick of the light. Still, it spooked me. Many years later, as building was taking place on the site of Nelly Cuckoo's cottage, there were some strange goings-on and a priest was brought in to bless the house. My brother erected a cross on the edge of the field, near the unmarked cemetery, to commemorate the dead and lay their souls to rest.

Daddy sometimes talked a bit when we sheltered from the rain in the cottage, recounting stories of the potato famine and hard times gone by. He was an amazing storyteller and poet who had a few dozen poems and madrigals at the tip of his tongue that he could recite with eloquent, dramatic flair. His children only very rarely got to hear or see him perform these gems. Some nights at home, however, when visitors came, and we all sat around the fire, toasting bread on a long fork, he launched into a historical ballad, a poem that seemed to go on forever or a memorised folk tale, and my little toes would curl with delight – my daddy, the reclusive, yet extraordinary, storyteller poet. He loved an audience, did Daddy, it was like two different people lived in the same man – the stern, strict, strong farmer and the consummate, compassionate, sensitive showman.

I loved his stories and I therefore loved when it rained in the Glebe. That said, Daddy had a real temper on him betimes. I can remember how angry he got when I broke the wooden connecting-rod on the grass-topping machine. That was a pet hate of his – as if I could see the bit of bog oak peeping up out of the soil in the long grass in time to slam the brakes on the tractor. I tried to reason with him that the rod was wooden because it was supposed to break if the bar got jammed and that that was a good thing – but as far as Daddy was concerned, clearly I should have had X-ray vision to detect all obstacles through the grass. The attainment of X-ray vision would prove an unspoken goal that I carried into my adult career as a surgeon to this day.

In time, I became quite a good tractor driver (in my own head, at least) and my confidence grew – too quickly, unfortunately! I never in my entire life heard my daddy utter the word 'fuck' – he was deeply religious and never cursed – that is, except on one fateful day in the Glebe. I was twelve years old, the summer between my childhood and my adolescence. We had just finished cutting the barley and it was all piled up in a several-ton trailer at the back of the tractor. The driver of the combine harvester was nowhere to be seen and in my infinite wisdom I thought that it would be most useful if I could drive the tractor out onto the lane and have it ready to go on its way to the grain depot. What I didn't account for, though, was that to drive a tractor and trailer out through a narrow gap, over a bridge, onto a lane, turning to the left, one should turn much wider, especially with a long-wheel axle trailer – much, much wider! Did I do that? Of course not! I turned short.

The trailer followed my short turning arc. The back wheel went up and then over the little cement ridge commonly found on farm bridges crossing streams. The tractor shuddered as the trailer was keeling over and I jammed on the brakes. The back axle went up on the side of the cement ridge. This stream was about 8 feet deep and 6 feet wide, but at that moment it may as well have been a gaping cavernous ravine that I was staring into, helplessly, from the tractor seat. My heart plummeted into that abyss. The trailer hovered and seesawed, perched precariously on the precipice – a giant barley-pendulum ready to swing and send the trailer and its load tumbling into the stream below. I was about to lose the harvest. I was going to be crucified.

I felt one side of the tractor begin to lift up. Then everything happened in slow motion. The tow bar locked on the link pin in the hitch on the back of the tractor, and all sorts of possibilities flashed through my head. Was the trailer going to rip off the chassis and tip over anyway? Was the tow bar going to warp and tip over anyway? Was the tractor going to turn and tip over anyway, bringing the trailer and its precious cargo downward? Each of these frantic, imagined outcomes ended in me, the tractor, the trailer and the barley harvest all tipping into the stream, though interestingly my imminent death wasn't among my imaginings. While my mind was thus occupied, to the left of my vision I saw the poor driver of the combine harvester trying to scramble back over a gate and simultaneously do up his trousers, after taking a call of nature in the next field. On my right, Daddy was running down the lane shouting, '*Holy blue fuck, Holy blue fuck!*' I had – and still have – no idea why 'fuck' was on that occasion 'blue', but I feared that I was going to be beaten black and blue.

At that moment, the combine harvester driver stumbled at the top of the gate and fell off it, with his trousers around his ankles. He scrambled to pull them up as he ran towards me and the teetering trailer, and both he and Daddy arrived at exactly the same moment. The trailer continued to seesaw. 'Grab the chain, Sean!' the driver shouted. Both seemed instinctively to know what to do. The combine driver ran to his machine and reversed it towards the tractor-trailer, while my dad grabbed a chain which was fortunately wrapped around the hitch at the back of the combine. Quick as a flash, he wrapped the chain around a flange at the back of the trailer and, when secured, he shouted to the combine harvester guy to pull. The combine moved forward a few feet, and the trailer stopped rocking. My heart had nearly stopped too as I got down out of the tractor cab. Once stabilised, they laid heavy-duty planks of wood under the trailer wheels and slowly crowbarred the trailer back up off the side of the bridge. By then, some help had arrived, and the combine pulled the trailer and the tractor backwards to safety. The barley had not crashed into the water below, but all of my tractor-driving confidence certainly had taken an almighty plunge.

Understandably, Daddy was absolutely livid. He never, ever beat or even hit me in his life, but I might have preferred that to the verbal lashing which lasted for days. Conversely, I can't remember him ever in my childhood actually saying the words '*sorry*' or, indeed, '*well done*', when I had actually done something right. I know he meant to say those things, as well as *'I'm proud of you'* and *'I love you'*, but his language was one of action rather than diction, and the action was that of a nod or a silent smile, rather than a slap on the back or a hug – that wasn't his way or the way of most Irish farmers at the time. So, at that time of my life, I didn't expect acknowledgement and didn't seek it, a trait I carry through to the present day.

Daddy didn't talk to me much about anything other than farming during my childhood or teenage years, though I know he was secretly proud, and Mammy told me since that he voiced this pride to others, just not directly to me. He had been much harder on my older brother than he had been on me, as he came from a culture where real men did not cry, real men got on with the job, real men did whatever was necessary and did not look for praise, acknowledgement or direct reward.

There is no question but that Daddy tried to look after me and my brother and sisters as best he could, both practically and financially. He paid the fees for clothes and books that I needed in secondary school, and he certainly helped me many times in university with money. There was one particular moment, though, when he gave me something entirely for the sake of giving, rather than the need to simply provide. It was my tenth birthday and I remember to this day the glint in his eye as he handed me a Timex wristwatch in a blue box. It had a round face and a brown strap. He just handed it to me in the hallway at our house, nodded and smiled. I opened it and, overjoyed, I went to hug him but he stepped back, just smiled again and was gone. Hugging was not really for him.

Mammy and Daddy absolutely loved all six children beyond doubt, but for them – and at that time in Ireland in general – hugging or kissing and physical demonstrativeness were simply not the done thing. It was just that as soon as we could stand on our own two feet, we were out on the farm and there was no encouragement for being a weakling or needing regular *plamasing* – as my parents put it – which meant in-gratiating flattery or cajoling. In my entire childhood, I only saw Mammy and Daddy hugging once in the kitchen, and that was by accident when I came in unexpectedly. I suppose they did it more regularly than I knew about – they did have six children after all – however, public displays of affection just weren't the code of conduct at the time.

Later in life, Daddy mellowed a bit and at least we had a bit more banter when I came home to visit. Ours was then more of a friendship than I'd ever had with him before and I'm really happy, looking back, that we had that chance to laugh and smile a bit more in the latter years of his life, long after I was no longer his 'boy on the farm' or his 'son who wanted to be a vet'. His aversion to hugging, however, remained. One day, after we got back from mass, where I had been 'out of order' in questioning parts of the Book of Genesis during the drive home, I went to give him a hug in the kitchen as a physical manifestation of my acquiescence to his intransigent point of view, even if I didn't believe in the 'fiery ball' of God's wrath. Daddy froze. He didn't know what to do with this display of affection and acknowledge-ment of respect for what he stood for, and what he believed in. I backed off. This is probably why I hug people so much nowadays. I guess I started to overcompensate later in life, but I also do believe in the power of *a proper hug* – I think that it's half of all healing, not of the body per se, but of the heart and soul.

While emotionally I'm quite different from my father – certainly more tearful and huggy – physically we are very similar, and I have that same attachment to the land coursing through my veins. When I first laid my eyes on the field and the broken-down farm buildings that were to become the veterinary practice now seen every week on *The Supervet,* I felt that same primordial connection. The moment I saw those derelict barns, I knew in a split second that this was my spiritual home and that I would do whatever it took to realise my dream there. I decided that I had to somehow make it mine, and then look after it, nurture it, and reclaim it, making it whole and teeming with animals once again.

When we were building Fitzpatrick Referrals, we couldn't change one inch of the outline as the land is in the protected greenbelt area. This, it transpires, was a good thing. I had found my oasis of calm, like Daddy and I had shared in the Glebe. I had found my own personal Glebe. Every day I feel extraordinarily fortunate to look out across the field at nature's changing seasons, though I'm quite sure that poor Daddy would be wide-eyed with shock if he knew how much I'd paid per square foot for it. Buying a home for Fitzpatrick Referrals was very far from the *sweet deal* that my father would have approved of, but needs must!

I am really glad that my daddy got to visit the practice once in his life, about halfway through its construction. He was all dressed up in his blue Sunday suit, walking around with his grey hair coiffed, his best handkerchief in his breast pocket and his hands behind his back like noble, landed gentry. It was clear to me, and to Mammy by his side, that he was proud, even if he never said it directly to me. I suspect there was always a little bit of him that was disappointed that I didn't stay in Ireland as a large animal vet, and a farmer. Still, I think I could see pride in his eyes and I was so grateful to have the opportunity to show him what I'd created here.

I wonder if it sank in when I told him that I had built one corner of the practice specifically for him. Everybody at the time, including the bank, said that my plan to build a cosy lecture theatre in the top end of the restored old hay barn wasn't a sensible use of space. Because it was deemed a re-build rather than a new build by the local authorities, we had to sand down the old rusty trusses that had been supporting the building and enclose them in the walls. I wanted this to be a place of inspiration and education, because that old disused barn was exactly the same type and shape as the hay shed at home in Ballyfin, where on some wonderful occasions my daddy had inspired and educated me.

If it rained during the harvesting of hay or silage, Daddy and I often sought shelter in the top of the hay shed beside our farmhouse, and that was the only place that my daddy ever gave me any sort of fatherly guidance, or words of wisdom. He was not an easy fellow to get along with a lot of the time. He was complicated; kind, considerate, harsh and irascible, all at once. He was extraordinarily sensitive in many ways, but only ever cried to himself. Lots of people didn't like him because he rocked boats – in other words, he spoke his mind and followed his heart, so while being true to himself, he could (and did) offend others. He was often grumpy to one, and then nice as pie to another, almost in the same breath. However, in those stolen moments, sheltering in the hay shed, he sometimes softened and occasionally gave me fatherly advice that has stayed with me to this day. He told me to row my own canoe and never to join in partner-ship with anyone. In fact, he said that one should never join with anyone except in prayer, because if things weren't going too well, one could always get up and leave. He said that as he was getting weaker I was going to get stronger, and I needed to learn that strength of mind was more powerful than strength of body. He told me to learn all that I could and that knowledge was never a load to carry as it weighed nothing, but was worth everything. He imparted sagacious words about never being attached to material things, and was then baffled when I asked how come he was so attached to the farm, the land and the animals. He just said, 'That's different. That's not attachment. That's a way of life.' I guess this has influenced my own perception of the practice, in that I'm not at all attached to any of it from a material perspective, and I don't consider my emotional attachment to the animals and the people as anything other than a way of life. It is my destiny, I suppose.

Some of my daddy's advice no doubt paid off. If I had taken a business partner, I probably wouldn't have been able to re-invest every penny I've ever earned into the business, since business partnerships generally require profit dividends. I would not have been able to fund scholarships across the globe that have spawned some beautiful human beings of whom I'm very proud, particularly from the Ohio State University and the University of Florida. I would also never have been able to do operations for free, from time to time, like those on a hedgehog, buzzard, penguin or the very deserving cat or dog. It's probably good to have a partner with whom to share risk and stress – but if I hadn't gone solo, as Daddy advised, Fitzpatrick Referrals probably wouldn't exist. I've taken some stupid risks and made some bad mistakes, but I did it on my watch and I did it my way. 'Thanks, Daddy – for the sound advice imparted as we stood out of the rain in that barn. Though there has been considerable hardship along the way, and even though, like you, I have started out with nothing at all, and it takes its toll, which is something you also know only too well, it has been worth it.'

Daddy was always a man of 'waste not, want not'. He reused the same piece of baler twine to hold up his trousers for years, and when it wore out and got too short, he used that same scrap of twine to tie up a gate instead of throwing it away. He was a hoarder of the highest order, and so am I. Well, if I wasn't, there's many an operation might fail as I wouldn't have a spare bit for it hidden away in Narnia – which is what we call the store cupboard in my office.

Daddy never really understood why I was motivated to do what I do, but he made me who I am and I wonder if he ever saw himself in me. Above all, he taught me to make the best of what I had, and to work hard. Many times in my youth, with sacks tied to our knees and shins with baler twine, Daddy and I would be hunched over all day, come rain or hail, crawling along the drills of soil to weed the turnips. Weeding the turnips, a boring, muddy, soggy job, was one of my very least favourite. I simply hated it. Every now and then I would accidentally pull up a baby turnip in my haste to pluck out the weeds, completely failing the objective of the exercise in the first place, which was of course to have a uniform row of fine turnips with no big gaps in the drills – a sinful waste of fertile soil. Daddy would momentarily stop, raise his head and look back at me with the muffled words, 'I heard that!' I wondered for years how it was that my daddy could hear a baby turnip being plucked out of the soil amid the pelting rain. Of course, what I only figured out a few years ago was that he couldn't hear anything. Instead he noticed me momentarily freezing to the spot after I'd plucked the turnip. In truth, by the end of a long day, I could barely see the difference between a baby turnip and a weed, my knees sore and my hands aching, but Daddy worked determinedly to finish the last few drills before nightfall, and so I silently suffered on – with only one or two notable exceptions. In my mind my daddy was the best turnip weeder ever to grace the face of the earth.

I remember one such evening quite vividly when, after an interminably long time as I wished for night to descend, I finally looked up and wailed, 'Daddy, my hands are full of thorns!' He paused for a brief moment, raised his head from the drills, looked back at me and said one single immortal line which has stayed with me forever since. 'Carry on, Noel – sure, when enough thorns have gone in, no more can get in. Carry on!' And so we did, we carried on.

My daddy taught me that hard work will get you anywhere you want to go, no matter how many pricks may get in your way. I internally repeated this aphorism many times later in life when I have faced adversity. I remember the thorns and I remember how many pricks need to go in before I begin not to feel the pain so much.

Now that I'm older, I realise that our lives have many parallels. Daddy started out with nothing and made his own way, by his own intelligence, determination, toil and sweat. This has been my experience too, and I have come to learn that the only thing worth having is what I earned myself. He was married to the land as I am married to my practice. He had farming running through his veins and my dedication to animals runs through mine. He never saw work as work, but just as a way of life. It's exactly that way for me too: being a vet has never been a job, but a vocation; never a chore, but always a privilege. I often think about this, especially if I have turned up late yet again to some dinner, social event or a date because I've been in theatre operating. As a vet,

I've never actually considered that I'm going 'to work' as a day job. Rather, I feel genuinely grateful to be a veterinary surgeon and to be allowed to do what I love to do every day of my life. In that, I know that I'm a very lucky man.

I have my daddy to thank for instilling his work ethic within me, for if he hadn't, I wouldn't be where I am today. Yet, in all of this, I'd like to think I've conditioned myself over the years to be conscious of my moods and temper, to control the irritability that comes from working crazy hours, together with the pressure of challenging surgeries and running a business. However, I'll be the first to admit that I don't always win in this pursuit, and I'm a right grumpy old badger some days. Sometimes it's because a client has really upset me, I've had a crisis of some kind with a colleague, an operation hasn't gone according to plan or because the bank, the lawyers and the clients are all hurling something at me at the same time, but mostly it's because people don't get the bigger picture – animals matter, people matter, and animals in the lives of people matter. I've definitely been guilty in the past of bringing negative emotions onto the prep-room floor with me, just like Daddy did on the farm, and it's probably because he lived, ate and breathed his vocation, just like I do mine. I'm getting better – I hope – because nowadays, I go upstairs to my bedroom and put my head on the pillow, breathe deeply and try to change the frame in the movie running through my head. I sometimes even say a prayer.

On 22 August 2006, I was working at the first Fitzpatrick Referrals premises, which was a hut surrounded by woods in Tilford in Surrey, when the phone call came to tell me Daddy was in hospital and it wasn't looking good for him. I ran from my office into the woods and as far as I could until there was darkness in the undergrowth, and there I fell on my knees, and I wailed. My hero was dying. I cried and cried until I could cry no more. I couldn't even begin to come to terms with this devastating news.

Daddy had been out at the back of our house, seeing to the cattle in the yard, when he suddenly collapsed. He was unconscious, and remained that way until he died a few days later. I got to his bedside at Portlaoise General Hospital – the very same place where I was born – and was crushed by a feeling of inadequacy. I had not been there to pick him up when he had fallen that day. I had failed. I held his hand and whispered into his ear, but I had – and still have – no idea if he heard me. I told him that I loved him very much, that I was very grateful for everything with which he had blessed me, and I thanked him for doing his best. On 25 August, Mammy said that she had noticed a 'change' in the afternoon, and he passed away two hours later. My daddy – that larger than life man whom I tried to emulate in so many ways – simply stopped breathing, my mammy holding his hand and his family all around him. He was eighty-two years old, but in my head and heart he was ageless, a small giant of a man, my daddy, my hero.

Mammy found Daddy's sudden death very difficult. She never got to say goodbye and she had desperately wanted him to tell her what to do with the stock and the farm. She had nightmares about it for years afterwards. Everyone grieves differently, but I know that for both Mammy and myself the healing tears didn't come until much, much later, and the empty space in our hearts was never to be filled. There was no definitive closure and no goodbyes, and sometimes I'll cry now for no apparent reason when I face some crisis or other, and I wish with all my being that I could talk with him.

Apparently, he had a brain haemorrhage and would have known nothing about it. He was lucky. This was exactly the way he wanted to go, to die working. Daddy never wanted to retire and he didn't want to die of illness or be a burden to anyone. I had been working toward my dream, as he wanted me to do, even if he never really understood what that dream was. I wish I could ask him what he thinks of what I'm doing now.

I hope that Daddy is somewhere in a parallel universe where there are lots of cattle and sheep to be minded and some bog land to be reclaimed. I wish I could say to him that I really respect him and I love him very much, even though we never actually said that to each other.

If I could speak to him now, there are many things I would say. I do understand why you couldn't pick baby Noel and Mammy Rita up from hospital. It was because your task in hand could not be successfully delegated to another. I too find it difficult to delegate the surgery, Daddy, but with you looking down on me, I think I'm getting better. If I'm ever lucky enough to have a baby of my own, I'll make sure that I am there at the birth and I'll think of you as I gently hug that precious little life. I'll close my eyes and imagine you saying to me, *I'm proud of you, Noel* – and I will say to you, *I'm proud of you too, Daddy*. I miss you, Daddy. You are always beside me in my head and in my heart.

CHAPTER THREE

The Robin and the Chestnut Tree

Childhood in Ballyfin

As soon as I could crawl, I was very quickly walking; as soon as I could walk, I quickly ran; and as soon, almost, as I could run, I was climbing trees. I loved to climb to the very highest branch I could reach in the big chestnut tree in the orchard out the back of our house. I always knew there was something else out there; I just had to climb high enough to see. I found an old log and hollowed it out to make a telescope, and perched it among the chestnut's branches to look out to far-and-distant places in my imagination.

One day a tiny red-breasted robin landed on the end of my telescope, and I dreamed of flying off with him and having adventures we could share. Peering through the pretend telescope, I imagined that I flew around the world accompanied by this Mr Robin, fixing all of the injured and sick animals. The animals sent me secret messages on leaves that only I could read, so that I could track them down and cure whatever was wrong with them – I suppose kind of like a fax from nature. Sometimes when I saw a leaf on the ground I imagined that it was another message from an animal somewhere far beyond our farm. Sitting up in my tree, I went on these fantastic adventures with Mr Robin, and when he flew away it was as if my dreams and hopes soared with him. This robin – or one of the relatives that looked just like him – came to visit me often, and I couldn't wait to get home from school to climb the tree and see if he would appear. Over the years, since my earliest encounters with Mr Robin, these familiar and sociable little birds have been an auspicious presence in my life, appearing to me at various, and strangely serendipitous, times as a sentinel of success, or as a saviour in times of fear and sadness.

Of course, I fell down from the branches often but that didn't stop me from getting back up and climbing to my hideaway in the sky again. Thankfully, I never suffered serious injury, but I sometimes think that maybe my early climbing years were formative in my choice to be an orthopaedic and neurosurgeon. While I was too young at the time to notice any such subliminal harbingers of the future, I have always been fascinated by the skeleton and the mechanics that control it, especially by the healing of bone – something that looks so inert on an X-ray picture, and yet has this ability to grow and to heal. As a child, I'd prod and poke my bruises with interest and I often watched my daddy repair the broken bones of lambs with splints that he cobbled together from sticks and baler twine. I thought this was a miracle.

I wanted to be able to fix bones and make them grow again. I had no idea at all how biology worked and didn't learn any such things at primary school. It was all a mystery, but an intriguing and fascinating one. I was growing up in a world where the animals and the farm were integral to the tapestry of my existence. There was no dividing line in my head between life and death, because I saw both on the farm.

However, it was suffering that hit me hard. Every time I saw an animal with a broken leg or in pain, I felt that pain on a deeply personal level and I didn't quite understand why. I just couldn't bear to witness any suffering in a living creature.

On the farm, there was a necessarily perfunctory attitude to animals. Every animal had a use and the sheep and the cattle clearly would not exist if it weren't for the meat and the milk they provided. At the end of the day, apart from our sheepdog and some farm cats, every animal I was herding, ministering to, dehorning, milking, shepherding, dosing, injecting, bedding, feeding or looking at was going to be eaten at some point. I never thought, or had reason to believe, otherwise in my childhood. I accepted this because it was part of me, genetically and environmentally. I saw the rabbits shot; I saw the rats and mice killed. When I was strong enough, I held the lambs as they were castrated and the noses of the cattle with tongs as Daddy sawed off their horns. I saw pigs pushed into milk churns, squealing as they had their testicles removed. I saw the lambs I helped to rear with a bottle get slaughtered, and the cattle herded with sticks and goads into trucks and taken to the meat factory never to be seen again. That was the way it was on our farm, and every farm at that time. This was my universe and this was my way of life. I even heard the sound of puppies being drowned by a man at a cattle mart once. I was very young at the time and this traumatised me more than I can actually express.

In a parallel universe, inside my head, there was a world where I saved all of the animals, no matter how broken or disfigured or abandoned. From a very early age, I had an idea that maybe someday I could be a vet, and I watched with fascination when our farm vet, Mr MacInerney, came out to treat the livestock. I was baffled, and hugely impressed, by how he knew which of the many bottles in the boot of his car to use. He would inject a magic potion into the vein of a cow and she would recover. I wondered if one day I might be able to do that.

I have four sisters and one brother. My three older siblings, John, Mary and Frances, were born in quick succession, each one year apart. After a five-year gap my sister Grace arrived, followed two years later by myself and, after another two years, my youngest sister, Josephine. We younger three attended primary school together, in a small, rural two-teacher school, called Barnashrone. It was just a few miles from where we lived, and it was a safe place. Weather permitting, we generally walked and in the winter the parents would organise a minibus to pick up children around the farms to take them to and from school.

Grace went off to secondary boarding school while I still had two years to go, and so it was just Josephine and me. We became the best of friends and the worst of enemies – sibling rivalry was at the core. We were once fighting over a coveted cattle stick: a carefully whittled sapling we used for herding cows. I was taunting her with it from inside Daddy's grey Morris Minor, poking it through the window at her. She grabbed it and, to prevent her thievery, I rolled up the window hard, trapping the stick, but also shattering the window into a million pieces in the process. Daddy was furious with us both, even though it was all my fault. On another day, we were forbidden to get out of that same car, which was parked a few feet away from O'Donaghue's shop in our local town, Mountmellick. We both sat trapped and yearning for the *Beano* comic that we could clearly see, tempting us with its free Gnasher glove puppet, attached to Dennis the Menace's mischievous face, on the cover. To my abject misery, Josephine was given the same prized comic book later that week and, to my eternal shame, I stole and stashed the puppet away out of sheer jealousy. Albeit illicitly acquired, this was my very first pet dog – a prize worth fighting for, I felt! I only finally fessed up to it a few years ago and have tried to make amends since, but I'm still not sure she has forgiven me.

Barnashrone Primary was a very small school. There were only three boys, including me, and three girls in my class, and about thirty-five students in total in the school. I was small of stature and wasn't particularly good at anything. I remember standing at the sidelines every time as the football team was picked. I never got picked except one time when one of the other boys was sick and, lo and behold, I scored a goal. That was the only great day I remember at primary school.

I started school in Barnashrone aged four, and during my first four of eight years there, I progressed well, but that was not my experience for the final four years when I switched to the second teacher. Primary school years are, educationally, the most formative years of any child's life, whereas I felt – and still do today – that I was horrendously short-changed during those precious years from eight to twelve years old. The days were mainly spent singing hymns and songs, saying the rosary, getting fuel for the classroom open fire and putting hot water bottles behind teacher's back. We did construct all manner of toys out of bits and bobs, but teaching in the core subjects of literacy and numeracy was hopelessly poor. Sadly, I came to realise that little of what I was taught there was either intellectually or practically useful. Corporal punishment was meted out for the smallest misdemeanour in the senior classes, and I was often the recipient of two or more whacks with a long, thin wooden stick. The most severe punishment of twenty strokes was inflicted on me for an alleged theft. We were asked to make small items of furniture from clothes pegs. Precision was always my strength and I had made a particularly good rocking chair. On the day that the varnish dried, I selected it from the windowsill to take it home. A class member insisted it was hers, and my teacher, without investigating the matter any further, called me to the front of the class and subjected me to the beating – twenty long hard strokes on the palms of my outstretched hands, ten on the left and ten on the right. I have never forgotten the injustice of that event.

As an adult, I am deeply saddened that my enduring memory of primary school is of injustice rather than the education I received. I was still writing – badly – on lined paper like an eight-year-old when I was twelve. The worst thing, looking back, was that I didn't know what I didn't know and I accepted it as the norm. Punishments were meted out in the name of God. The patronage and authority in the school were religious, yet I can't remember such behaviour ever being questioned. Nobody, including my parents, questioned it. It just wasn't the thing to do. Some things happened at that time in the name of God and the Church that are best forgotten.

Educationally, I was not set up well at all by my primary schooling. Whether this served me later by pushing me harder to catch up, or whether it was a hindrance, is hard to say, but it made my path through secondary school and thereafter a lot more challenging. One tangible consequence is that my handwriting remains diabolical to this day.

Mammy's mother, Annie, came to live with us at the farmhouse in 1972, after my grandad John died. She was a very elegant lady whom we cared for until the end of her life. We'd come home from school, eat dinner and then kneel down with Mammy and Granny to say the rosary prayer, as was the practice in many Irish Catholic homes at the time. We then had our chores to do, getting in turf for the fire or attending to the many jobs around the farm.

There was also no particular emphasis on acquiring any ancillary life skills in most rural households, in Ireland, in the 1970s. I look now at friends taking their children to karate, guitar, swimming, dance and football classes and I really do wish I'd had chances like that. We did go to a few swimming classes, but I was terrified and no effort was put into making it otherwise for me, so I am a poor swimmer to this day. I would have loved to go to drama classes but such a thing wasn't on anyone's priority list.

I loved comic books, which were full of pictures and not many words and suited my limited reading skills. I kept a secret stash of them under my bed, and in my pink wooden cupboard. I got them either by saving money gleaned from helping farmers at the cattle market, or by going to the 'bring and buy' comic-book sales that were periodically held at the school. Well, to be honest, I thought that my comics were secret, but when Josephine was old enough she covertly snaffled them. When I found out, I was livid but thankfully she was mainly interested in the *Beano* and *Dandy*.

My favourite was Marvel Comics' *The X-Men* – 'The Strangest Superheroes of all!' – featuring Wolverine, though I also loved DC Comics' *Batman with Robin The Boy Wonder*. I was a big fan of all the comic superheroes, and especially those who could miraculously heal their skeletons – or fly! I knew that both Batman and Wolverine felt different from all the world around them. Neither felt understood. Batman spent his life in search of the love he lost when his parents were murdered, while Wolverine was a mutant with a metal endoskeleton, and he had the ability to heal himself. I escaped into the comic books because I dreamed of a world where superheroes saved the day. In my daydreams, when Mr Robin and I flew from the chestnut tree, there were often some of my favourite comic-book superheroes alongside us. Batman was an obvious companion for my Mr Robin, but Wolverine and some of his pals often came too, since together we had our powers to heal – and to me, that seemed like the most amazing gift of all.

The reality of life on a farm in Ballyfin was a far cry from Gotham City, however. There were cattle and sheep to look after, sheds to be bedded with straw, muck to be scraped off yards, turnips to be weeded, silage and hay to be cut, barley to be harvested, and so on: the endless cycle of work with each changing season. Along with weeding the turnips, some of my least favourite jobs were cleaning the yards, oiling the cattle cubicles and picking stones. Cleaning the yards involved taking a scooper-scraper behind a tractor and driving the excrement up a ramp and into a slurry tank. Years later, I was working as a vet on a farm where a fellow had actually died doing this because the tractor turned over into the tank. A horrible way to die, and being drowned in slurry is the cause of a recurring nightmare I suffer to this day.

Oiling the cattle cubicles was an excruciatingly boring task, especially in the height of summer. In the yards, where they lived in winter, the cattle ate preserved grass from the face of a silage pit – which was a big mound of grass preserved between two retaining walls, and covered in polythene plastic – or were fed from a trough of grain nuts, and they would sleep in cubicles separated by metal railings. In the summer, we had to scrape all of the caked-on muck off the railings, and then clean them with wire brushes and paint them with the burned oil from the sump of the tractor engine.

Picking stones I especially loathed. After ploughing and tilling, stones had to be picked from the fields. This involved a very tedious process of walking endlessly and erratically behind a tractor that was moving very slowly in front, with a big metal transport box hooked to its rear, and gathering and throwing the stones into this large receptacle. For a while, when I was very young, I got to drive the tractor because I was too small to carry many big stones. This aspect of the labour was grand, as driving a tractor in a straight line was easy, but I was much resented by my older siblings. Finally, though, when I was big enough, I too had to be in the 'picking-up posse', toiling for days on end in the stony ground, which was no fun at all.

I learned how to turn the tractor eventually, and in the end became reasonably adept at it – apart from the time I nearly upended the barley crop into the river – and so I got the job of rolling the soil. Behind the tractor was the roller, a huge metal cylinder on an axle, which was intended to level out the ground and knock down any residual stones into the soil before planting grain seed, so that the harvester wouldn't pick up stones and soil later on. I had to simply drive the tractor with the roller in a straight line to one end of the field, turn around and drive back in an equally straight line. I prided myself on my precision, but I was also very small, and one day a neighbour, Mrs Coleman, phoned my mother at home in a state of great distress to tell her that the tractor was driving itself around the field. There was no sign of my little head above the steering wheel!

Other farm jobs were potentially fun, such as drawing

hay and silage, and dipping sheep. They were actually social events in that all our relatives, friends and passers-by got roped in to help. The objective of sheep dipping, which usually happened twice in the summertime, was to rid the sheep of external parasites such as blowfly, lice, ticks and scab, which could result in major health problems. It was the most spectacular mayhem. All the sheep were corralled into a pen and then ushered, or more correctly flung, into a giant channel of water with sheep-dip solution in it. Pandemonium and frivolity and the putrid water flowed in equal measure, as human bodies flailed everywhere, amid crazy sheep, slipping and sliding. The poor animals hated it and were scared – literally – shitless. Poo emanated from every direction as they were flung into the giant bath of dip treatment and had to swim to the other side to clamber out. If they hadn't had enough of a dipping, Daddy, or another helper, would hold the exit gate and push them back down under the surface with a big Wellington-booted shove. Everyone was soaked but in good spirits, cheered by the circus-like performances of the handlers, as at the time it was fun for almost all concerned – except the sheep, poor creatures. The fun for many farmers throughout the country was short-lived, though, as quite a number were affected by organophosphate poisoning from the sheep-dips widely available in Ireland in the seventies and eighties. Some of those chemicals were of the same group from which chemical warfare agents are developed. They contaminated soil and waterways in some cases and also caused cumulative toxicity in some farm workers for years after exposure. Sometimes there is regress as well as progress in animal care, a theme which would echo in my later life.

There were other episodes of bona fide fun in my childhood

and not all were related to farm work. I did get to go to Irish dancing in my little brown first Holy Communion suit, along with Grace and Josephine in their lovely green embroidered dresses, and I was an altar boy who assisted at mass, which I enjoyed. Indeed, I would become the longest-serving altar boy – to my knowledge – in the history of Ballyfin Church. I liked the ceremony of the role, though it was also a source of much-needed revenue for me to subsidise the occasional comic, sweets or my summer holiday money. Further, I got to dress up, and I had a certain amount of power carrying the thurible full of incense. This was a golden metal censer suspended from chains that the altar boy gently swung to keep it burning, until the priest took it and vigorously swung it over something holy, or in a gesture of affirmation as the prayers of the faithful rose on the mist towards heaven. I was good at this job, except on one occasion when the soporific incense made me fall asleep and I fell over on the step in front of Father Moran.

On another occasion, I almost got excommunicated. During one particularly long and boring sermon, I was sitting on the step in front of the pulpit at Father Moran's socked feet encased in his sandals, when, for some reason, I got it into my head that I would be able to reach out really slowly and surreptitiously touch his big toe. As the tips of my fingers got within an inch of the priest's sock, I got the most almighty kick, which sent my hand reeling. I whimpered internally as the sermon carried on, and I thought I'd be lynched. Instead he just looked at me knowingly and, if looks could kill, I'd be six feet under. Since that day, I have forever hated sandals with socks.

The most challenging and prestigious job for an altar boy, however, was carrying the cross as we processioned around the Stations of the Cross at Easter time. No server earned money for this, but it built arms of steel and often gained points with Father Moran. If the cross didn't shake at all during the procession, while the cortege stopped for prayers at each of the fourteen stations which mapped the passion and death of Christ, then maybe he might let you sit by the coffin at the next funeral – and that was a financially rewarding activity. I was always very sad when we got to the bit where Jesus was crucified, but remarkably I cheered up no end at the prospect of the next funeral when I'd be next to the coffin, and therefore get the biggest tip from the mourners. Weddings were the other major source of income. I was fantastic at looking sad or happy as the moment demanded at funerals or weddings.

My ability as an altar boy must have impressed our new parish priest, Father Meaney, as he fed me Latin books in the hope that he had a vocation on his hands. He and my mammy had several conversations about whether I would have potential for the priesthood. Years earlier, when I was with my godmother, Mrs Dunne, who lived right beside the church, she looked out at the venerable building and asked whether I'd like to wear 'the big vestments' in there one day – by which it was obvious, even to me, she meant the clothes of the priest. I just looked at her, in my innocence, and said that I'd probably never be big enough to grow into them. She didn't raise the subject again, even after I was more than big enough, and I was still serving mass when I had vastly outgrown my surplice and my soutane vestments. Father Meaney actually offered me his vestments if I would continue serving longer. I never really seriously considered a religious vocation because, although I absolutely believe in a spiritual connection through all things, which is God I suppose, I had trouble with the Adam and Eve bit and the bit about the fiery flames of hell. I did like serving mass, though. The ritual, order, predictability and certainty it entailed was reassuring in my teenage years, in the midst of what would become an uncertain life at secondary school. Furthermore, as an altar boy, I was acknowledged and praised, which was something that didn't happen often in real life.

As an altar boy, I got to go to the old folk's party at Ballyfin Community Centre, as a special dispensational treat. I was a big hit with all of the ladies of a certain age with whom I danced and waltzed and, most importantly, after each dance I got a prized Club Milk biscuit. I was by no means a good dancer, but in such company I was considered nimble and thus my Irish dancing prowess served me well to snaffle my bellyful of Club Milks which, to me at the time, were the Holy Grail of confectionery.

Confectionery, mostly baked by Mammy, was also in plentiful supply at my birthday parties. Mammy always put in a real effort every year baking a fantastic cake and loads of iced buns. Mammy was the best baker in all of Ireland in my opinion, and iced currant cakes were her speciality. My two classmates, Larry Walsh and Terry Moore, were always in attendance. We'd play games like musical chairs and hide-and-seek. It was a highlight of the year for me because, at most other times, it was mainly work and not much play. Even the distance from their houses to mine, at that time, seemed enormous and so playing wasn't a daily occurrence, but birthdays were different. On the evening of a birthday I didn't have to do any chores; I could eat and play myself into oblivion.

The ultimate highlight of the year for me, however, was the

much-anticipated family trip to Tramore, a seaside resort in County Waterford, where we rented a caravan for two weeks every summer. I saved up all the money I earned from getting in sheep for Mr Lewis, our neighbour across the fields, and serving as an altar boy and stashed it in a silver Ovaltine tin. This was carefully stored in the drawer of the pink wooden cupboard in my room, along with other treasures like my favourite key rings, comics and any chocolate bars or sweets that I managed to purloin during Lent. I had made a lock for the drawer to keep Josephine out of it. All through Lent, as I craved the chocolate bars, I occasionally looked into the drawer to check my stash, and I would gingerly open up the Ovaltine tin and check how much I had for the faraway paradise of Tramore that summer. For the forty days and forty nights of Lent, from Ash Wednesday to Easter Sunday, Father Moran said that mortifying the flesh and self-denial were the way forward for repentance of sins and the pathway to heaven, but, to be honest, Tramore was the heaven in my head at that time.

When the day to go to Tramore finally arrived, Mammy, and whichever children were in the mix at that time, all piled into our grey Morris Minor with Daddy in the driver's seat. There could be up to nine people in that tiny Morris Minor. Three adult children with siblings of various sizes on their knees squeezed up on the back seat, while Mammy sat in the passenger seat with another small child perched near the gear stick. I guess there were very few observed rules of the road in Ireland in the 1970s! A bag of potatoes was generally shoved under Mammy's feet in the front, along with various other bits and pieces, such that her legs were up in the air; the car boot was similarly packed with buckets and spades and clothes and various accoutrements of holiday travel.

The pram was strapped to the back. One time, we pulled up at our destination, much to the amusement of a passer-by who delivered a running commentary of, 'Oh my goodness, there's another one coming out!'

One year, I was so excited that I jumped out of the car, ripped off my shoes and ran off down the beach as quickly as my little legs could carry me, only to slash my foot on a big bit of glass hidden in the sand. I was crying and Daddy carried me off to the doctor to get it stitched up. Daddy drove us all to Tramore, but summer being a very busy season on the farm, he generally only stayed for a couple of days at a time – driving up and down the eighty miles to and from Ballyfin long before there were motorways – in order to give his family an annual holiday. The time of his departure or arrival was generally very late at night. I remember once turning up at the caravan at midnight with him after harvesting silage all day, which I had stayed on at home with him to do. To Daddy, time was a continuum – day and night didn't matter. Another time, he turned up unexpectedly and my sister Frances's boyfriend, Liam, who was not supposed to be in the caravan, had to get out of the back window sharpish!

Throughout my childhood, Daddy rarely took more than a few days off each year, and when he did, he was always worried about what was happening back home so he'd walk to the phone in the kiosk at the middle of our caravan park to call whoever was looking after the cattle and sheep and ask them long and detailed questions. I wouldn't have wanted to be in their shoes if anything had gone wrong. To this day, I guess I lick my paucity of holidays from the same bowl as Daddy, and if I go off lecturing, I'm on the phone and answering emails all of the time. If I took an actual holiday, I would probably be like him, too. In Tramore he'd sleep for the first day of his holiday, which generally left him only one day to rejoice in his 'relaxed' state by walking down the promenade like a man of veritable leisure and money – neither of which was true.

Our holiday in Tramore was an epic journey of adventure and possibility, though. There was sand on which to build castles, sea in which to paddle, other children to befriend and, most importantly, an amusement arcade. This was a spectacular, gaudy, phantasmagorical wonderland full of fairground rides to go on and machines where, if you put in a penny or two pence, you might just win a fortune. It was for these extraordinary adventures that I saved my hard-earned money, and when it came to spending it, I considered very carefully where, and planned exactly how much I could spend each day, to extend my stash of cash from the Ovaltine tin to the very last day of the holiday. Usually I had about two pounds for each day. There was always the vague hope that I might win some money on the amazing Penny Falls machine, where you'd put in a coin and, if you timed it correctly, you could knock lots of others off the ledge and into a winnings tray – but I never did.

I knew nothing of the world before age eleven, other than from our annual trip to Tramore – I had only ever been to Dublin less than a handful of times. The furthest I could think of, or imagine, was what I had seen on our black-and-white television set. This was powered by a coin box that took fifty-pence pieces, the mechanism for paying the rental fee at the time.

Whenever I wanted to watch television, I could always earn fifty pence somehow, either by getting in sheep for our neighbour Mr Lewis, helping with some cattle loading or assisting at the weekly Wednesday market in Mountrath. I could watch until the fifty pence in the box ran out, though I have to say I actually don't remember watching anything, when I was very little, except *Sesame Street*. I was intrigued by the cultural diversity, because where I lived in Ireland there was none. That was the first place I saw children who looked different from my family and community. I particularly enjoyed the game 'One of These Things is Not Like the Others', because I didn't know whether they were referring to the colour of the hats the children were wearing or the actual children themselves. I was an innocent seven-year-old in a cultural bubble – Ballyfin at the time certainly wasn't exactly the epicentre of societal or ethnic diversity. As with the paucity of education at school, I just didn't know what I didn't know.

I existed in total ignorance about the world in general until the late seventies, when I was about ten or eleven years old. It was at this time too, that two characters came into my life through that old black-and-white television, that made me question the status quo. The first was the Six Million Dollar Man. Steve Austin, for me, was a fantastical hero who, in the TV show at least, was bionic. He was stronger, faster, better than any human being. I wanted to be all of those things and more – yes, I wanted to be bionic, but I also imagined other possibilities in making animals and humans bionic. My dream was crystallised in the summer before I started secondary school when I went fishing on the River Shannon with my Uncle Paul.

Uncle Paul had had his leg amputated in a motorbike accident and everyone knew he had a wooden leg, but I had never actually seen it. It was a very hot day. In fact, one of the very few very hot days that I can remember in my childhood and Uncle Paul drove me forty-five miles or so to Athlone, a large town on Ireland's premier river, the Shannon. He was grumbling a bit towards the end of the journey, which wasn't usually in his character. I remember that his limp was getting limpier and his manner a bit grumpier as we got our fishing rods from the car boot, paid our fishing licence, hired a little blue boat and set off on our fishing expedition. We had only been out on the river for about ten minutes when the reason for his irritability became apparent. What happened next is lodged in my memory forever – in slow motion. Uncle Paul rolled up one of the legs of his trousers and, for the very first time, I saw his wooden leg. I was rowing with all my might and paused momentarily. Then he rolled his trouser up even further, revealing the straps that were holding his leg on. He undid the straps, huffing and puffing as the sun beat down from the bright blue cloudless sky. Little boats passing left and right with people fishing for trout took no notice, but I was transfixed. I was rowing and holding my breath all at the same time. Then suddenly and without warning he whipped the leg off. I stared in shock.

His stump looked like someone had taken a hammer to a side of bacon and bludgeoned it. It was horrible, smelly, scabby and oozy. The ill-fitting socket of his wooden leg had rubbed and chafed his poor stump. I was stunned. It was truly awful. No wonder he was a bit grumpy, I thought. As he let out a sigh of temporary relief – the likes of which I'm sure would be difficult to comprehend unless one had to put up with that pain all of the time – I let out a stifled scream.

At that very moment of my scream, I must have simultaneously dropped my oar from its ring and it flipped forward, catching Uncle Paul's false leg, which he had perched on the side of the boat, knocking it overboard. Oh my God; as it floated off downstream on the current, I thought I was going to be killed. Actually, Uncle Paul was remarkably sanguine about it. We just rowed off downstream, in pursuit, hoping it wouldn't end up in the Atlantic Ocean, as the smiles of happy fishermen with trout in their boats rowed by. No trout in our boat, and no smiles on our faces, we caught up with the leg a couple of hours later in the arms of an American tourist who was standing in a bed of reeds.

'*Anyone's leg? Anyone's leg?!*'

Yes – that will be ours!

As we spent the rest of the day rowing back upstream, there wasn't much said, so I had plenty of time to wonder why Uncle Paul didn't have a bionic leg fitted to his skeleton like Steve Austin. I didn't ask; it wasn't the moment.

The idea of becoming a vet had crystallised after the loss of those very first two lambs in a frozen field, but after witnessing Uncle Paul's distress that afternoon in the boat I was determined that one day I would find out how to put on a bionic leg. I just thought it was utterly stupid that poor old Uncle Paul had to put up with all that pain, infection and inconvenience. I did know that Steve Austin wasn't really bionic – but surely it was possible, I thought. Stronger, faster, better. This would be my goal.

The second, seminal discovery I made through our TV set was of a new hero who inspired a whole world of possibility in my mind. He was a role model for me because he defied all of the odds to triumph. Alongside Batman, Wolverine and the Six Million Dollar Man, he was almost more important, because he was actually real; well, real in a movie anyway. Back then, in 1979, I didn't go to a cinema, as that was practically unheard of for a child at primary school in Ballyfin. However, I had heard all about the *Rocky* movie and I knew that Raidió Teilifís Éireann (RTÉ) was going to show it on the television, so I saved up fifty-pence pieces in my Ovaltine tin. I was beyond excited as the day arrived and the coins kerchinged into the box and the television burst into life. I snuck in behind the old flowery sofa in the living room, so that if Daddy came in to ask me to go out to the sheep, I would be nowhere to be seen.

I almost couldn't breathe in anticipation, as the theme music began. I huddled riveted, living every moment and completely awestruck when it came to the now-iconic scene where Rocky runs up the steps of the Philadelphia Museum of Art. The everyman was about to become a superman. A dream was about to be realised against all of the odds. Then, about half an hour before the end of the movie, the television died: I had run out of fifty-pence pieces. I was gutted. I had to wait to see the ending another day, but from that night Rocky was my definitive real-life hero and I yearned to go to Philadelphia. In fact, I yearned to go anywhere, and far away with Mr Robin by my side on fabulous adventures that were waiting for me outside my childhood and outside Ballyfin, beyond even the most distant hills that I could see from the top of our chestnut tree.

CHAPTER FOUR

The Cat and Her Kittens

My Mammy, Rita Fitzpatrick

She was scrawny, underfed and more than a bit wild when she turned up on our farm. Her orange-and-white fur was matted, and was home to a family of fleas. She was a feisty cat, but she would let me stroke her when nobody was watching. The cat was tolerated by Daddy because she caught mice, and then, when I was about eight years old, she gave birth to a litter of six kittens inside a hole in the straw bales where she had burrowed. Each night for about four weeks, after the cow in the shed out the back of our house had been milked, I siphoned off some of the warm frothy milk from the top of the bucket in the yard, and squirrelled it away in an old metal bowl for the kittens. When the kittens left their nest in the straw, for the first time in my life I genuinely felt that I had achieved something worthwhile.

I had great difficulty reconciling myself to the hierarchy of the animal kingdom. Over a year earlier, I had almost lost my life trying to scoop a mouse out of a grain silo. I felt so sorry for it scrambling to get up out of the big metal vat that I climbed in and helped him out, but I started to be sucked down into the grain and couldn't get any grip on the slippery sides with my little hands. Luckily a neighbour helping us with the harvest grabbed me out by the arm. Unluckily, just as the mouse jumped out, the neighbour squashed it with his big boot, saying that I was stupid and that he would teach me the order of things. I did understand what he was saying – but his words about 'the order of things' has stuck with me and shapes me to this day in terms of how I feel about our responsibility to the world of animals. Even though the cat's job was to kill mice, I guess I felt it was my job to look after *all* the animals – even the ill-fated mouse stuck in the silo.

My mammy absolutely knew the hierarchy and order of things in her life. The children always came first, all six of us. Daddy thought he was the boss in our house, but Mam knew better. She let him believe it was him making the decisions, but everyone knew where the seat of power really lay. Like the mother cat I looked after in the shed, she had built a safe home for all of her children, but was often left alone with the babies as Daddy went to fairs in distant counties. She was determined and resourceful, yet not proud and only had one vocation: to look after her brood of six, all of whom she loved and appreciated equally. Every time I talk to her about any achievement or milestone in my life, she reiterates this equitable sharing of her love. Conversely, I am of course completely biased – my mammy is the person I love most in the entire world.

Rita Keegan was born on 25 May 1929 in Ballina, County Mayo. She had a tough childhood. The Second World War broke out when she was only ten years old and rationing and gas masks arrived in the Republic of Ireland, as they did across the United Kingdom. The year 1939 was hugely significant in the Keegan family as it was for the whole world. Her father, John, lost his job in the hardware shop in Ballinasloe, along with the house attached to that position, and so the family was separated. Mammy's mother Annie brought the younger members of the family, Phil, Sean and Pat, to live with her sister in County Offaly, while John brought daughters Rita and Marie and son Tom to live with his sister Sarah in Dublin.

Dublin was about sixty miles away, but at that time, of course, and even in my childhood, the city seemed like a world away on a long and winding road. Mammy was a shy, sensitive ten-year-old and suddenly found herself in an alien school in Haddington Road, with people who indeed considered her alien. The other girls bullied her and ridiculed her country accent and lack of learning. She felt lonely and lost. It's probably no coincidence that, many years later, I was in the same boat at school. History has a habit of repeating itself with the sensitive ones.

In 1940 Mammy went back to Mayo to stay with family friends, and decided that Dublin was not for her, so she never returned. She made the best of what she had in a very difficult time and place. In fact, throughout her life, money was by no means flush; she often had to make the best of what she had, and recycle what she had not. John emigrated to England to work, while Annie with other members of the family rented a very small house in Mountmellick and also made the best of it. John sent home three pounds a week to the family, which they lived on together with a basic 'children's allowance' from the government.

Rita returned to Mountmellick aged thirteen and attended St Mary's secondary school, where all subjects were taught in Gaelic. As she had no foundation in the language she found school very difficult. On the bright side, however, she discovered a local drama group, and with some friends managed to learn a little Gaelic. Very soon, her main priority became dancing, particularly the three- and the eight-hand reels. She even occasionally won competitions, and when given the choice between a medal or a 'few bob', most of the time she took the money, which was only a few pennies but was far more useful than a silver medal in her poor circumstances. She saved this up to go to more dances.

She does, however, still have two glistening silver medals, which she and her friends won at the Feiseanna, where they put on a show and had to answer questions in Gaelic. Her life slowly improved, and when her father eventually came back from England, unfortunately crippled with arthritis, the family moved to an upstairs apartment on that same Mountmellick street, which was at least a proper home. I remember this house vividly, since most Sundays, as a small child, I visited my maternal grandparents John and Annie who still lived there, and it was here, I think, that some of my formative ideas as a surgeon took shape.

Indeed, my earliest childhood memory is of foraging in the big mahogany cupboard in their living room amid myriad tin cans, searching for the Holy Grail. These were small pieces of Meccano that had accumulated there over the years – probably from the previous tenants. The little metal pieces were earnestly ferreted out from cracks in the wooden base of the cupboard by my agile four-year-old fingers, every single piece like a nugget of gold, and used to build whatever came into my head. Mostly, however, my creations were only partially realised, because there weren't enough parts, so basically I'd build half of my dream creature and the rest existed in my imagination alone, as I flew a bionic bird high above a castle of tin cans, or a bionic bull charging at the cans and knocking them down. The bird might have wings, but no head and half a tail, and the bull have horns and a head, but no body. None of that mattered, because in my head they were fully-fledged, magnificent animals charging and flying around Granny and Grandad's living room on a Sunday afternoon. For many subsequent Christmases, Santa miraculously gifted me with more wonderful pieces of Meccano, and my lifelong obsession with plates and screws, and nuts and bolts was ensured.

After leaving school, aged fifteen, my mammy took an apprenticeship at Mrs Shortall's drapery shop in Mountmellick. She worked for no wages at all for two years to 'learn the trade.' This was basically where she and her lifelong friend, Sheila Egan, learned how to stitch hems in skirts, make tablecloths and sheets, modify garments of every shape and size and, most importantly, how to sell all manner of clothes, material, rugs and accessories associated with the drapery business. She was told she was useless and sacked almost daily by Mrs Shortall if she allowed a prospective customer to leave without buying anything.

This was Mrs Shortall's cardinal rule: never to allow any customer to leave without parting with some cash. Mrs Shortall herself was a par excellence specialist in retail extortion of the financially unwary. There was many the man or woman who came in only to browse and who left the shop with new shoes, a scarf or a belt, or indeed all three. There was a great focus on millinery and mantles – which are hats and coats to you and me. The girls were encouraged to chat to everyone in this artful wooing of the potential purchaser. All of the young men from the region came into the shop, asking them to get up and take various items down off 'the lines' – the wooden beams from which some products were suspended – just so that they could see the girls, of course!

One man asked what such and such an item on the beam was, and upon being told that they were pyjamas, he asked what such an item of clothing was for. My mother told him they were clothes for night-time, to which he retorted, 'Well I won't be needing them then, because I never go anywhere at night!' Another man, embarrassed at having to buy a corset for his wife who had just given birth (which was apparently the norm at the time), was stuttering and stammering when my mother established, only after persistent questioning, that he was looking for a 'belly-leveller'!

Mrs Shortall's girls were artists of retail chit-chat and masterminds of retail conversion. These formidable saleswomen, of course, learned every mandatory nuance of a transaction from the queen of drapery seduction, Mrs Shortall herself. She once sold my mother's brother Sean, when he was very drunk and very much a bachelor, three ladies' neck scarves, before sending him on his way. She had no mercy. You came in through the door and you went out with a purchase: that was the drill.

There were only a few exceptions to Mrs Shortall's rule of sell, sell, sell, and these were either with the very strong-willed or the extraordinarily drunk. One such drunkard, mistaking the door of the drapery store for Flannagan's public house next door, and the window alcove for the urinal, began to undo his zipper to relieve himself. Mammy told him in no uncertain terms to take himself and his 'business' elsewhere. The other extreme was my daddy, Sean Fitzpatrick. He was a 'pioneer' – he wore a pioneer badge affiliated with the Catholic Church indicating that he didn't drink alcohol at all, ever. This was naturally a major attraction to my mammy, whose father and brothers were seasoned drinkers, but she certainly played hard to get and if she did, he remained staunch, even when faced with Mrs Shortall. He came into the shop often, always on the pretence of bringing a message to Sheila Egan, who was his cousin, and took these opportunities to praise my mother loudly to whichever poor lad he brought in as a sidekick, mostly saying that my mam was a lovely girl – well within her earshot, of course. On a few occasions, he tried on shoes ostensibly to buy, but Mammy knew there was no way he had any intention of making a purchase; he was just eyeing her up. Daddy was a cattle dealer and a shrewd operator, so Mrs Shortall could not intimidate Sean Fitzpatrick, try as she may.

It was just as well that Daddy didn't drink alcohol because many farms were lost across a bar table in Ireland down through the years, and he would go in and settle all of the cattle buying and selling accounts in the pub. There were two pubs near Mrs Shortall's drapery shop and cattle dealers and cattlemen of all kinds were regulars in her shop. As in many Irish towns, the cattle were ushered into the high street and tied to various stalls here and there on fair day. Needless to say, the street was littered with bovine excrement, or cow shit, depending on your linguistic sensibilities, and the atmosphere was one of general mayhem. One day, a horned cow of some description charged through the narrow door of the drapery shop and Mammy and Sheila had to get up on the counter and hush it out with skirts, sheets, scissors and whatever else came to hand.

On one fateful night, in a dance hall some distance from Mountmellick, Sean Fitzpatrick finally asked Rita Keegan to dance. She said, 'No thanks. I'm all right,' but he walked her home anyway – his bicycle clips around his trouser legs – all the way to the door of her house, about ten miles away, and then cycled another five miles home. Love was in the air for Sean Fitzpatrick.

However, it wasn't love, but dancing that remained Mammy's main obsession in those years. She went to her drama and dancing classes at every available opportunity. Probably my leaning towards drama stemmed from her, but unlike Mammy, who wanted to dance because she didn't want to be standing around with two left feet, I didn't do so well in that department. In my childhood Irish dancing classes, I did my best, but I was no Michael Flatley. My mam, on the other hand, became a great dancer and once the drapery job offered her half-a-crown a week in her third year, she could afford a shilling and three pennies to go to the 'Cinderella' dance from 8.30 to 11.30 p.m. on a Tuesday night in the Owness Hall in Mountmellick.

Soon she was dancing all over the place at ceilis with her eight-hand reel, and even at the big band nights – waltz, foxtrot, quickstep, and tango. She still had to scrimp and scrape, though, to get to the dance. She and my dad's cousin, Sheila, even had to cut a headscarf in two, and each wear half, because they couldn't afford one each. They were no Cinderellas, however; in their minds they were fully-fledged dancing queens.

Sean Fitzpatrick persisted in his pursuit of his 'lovely girl', and I suppose he knew that he was in with a chance when one night she kissed him before going into her parents' house. He eventually got invited in to have cocoa with her mum and dad. In fact, John Keegan, Mammy's dad, had many years previously gone to school with my father's dad, Martin, meaning the future in-laws were already warmed up. Before long, Daddy flung caution to the wind and just went for it. He eventually asked their permission to marry Rita before asking Mammy herself. Mrs Shortall was the only one who was upset, because when Dad popped the question over Christmas in 1955, she had to give my mammy the day off to go to Dublin to get the engagement ring in McDowell's jewellers. However, they say that every cloud has a silver lining, and this was true for Mrs Shortall, at least. Daddy was by now a dapper fellow – he had a Morris Minor car at the time and a very flash Crombie coat. He was making an impression and becoming a respected cattle dealer, so the engagement ring was a stunner. Mrs Shortall was initially displeased that one of her best sales ladies was engaged, as she would cease to work there after the marriage. However, she finally saw the union in a most positive light because there were lots of folks coming into the shop to look at the ring and, as a result, hats and scarves were flying off the shelves to those willing to buy in the haze of my parents' impending marital bliss.

Of course, nothing could be further from the truth. My Mammy and Daddy were mostly happy enough and certainly did love each other, but this marriage, like relationships the world over, was to be no walk in the park. They tied the knot on 24 September 1956 in Mountmellick with forty people in attendance. Remarkably, Mrs Shortall got her daughter, Patricia, to drive my mam and herself to Dublin to help her to choose a wedding dress of appropriate cloth and calibre, and subsequently confided in her niece, Maura Wolfe, that Rita 'was a nice honest girl' and that 'she had always been her favourite'! She even took her to Arnotts department store – one of the leading Dublin drapery stores – to help her to buy a 'going-away dress' for the honeymoon. Finally, the years of servitude resulted in the acquisition of some superior-quality sartorial elegance for Rita herself.

What followed were two weeks of honeymoon driving around the south of Ireland, the last stop carefully planned in a fashion prescient of things to come – it was in Waterford so that Daddy could get to the cattle fair on time. Such was his life: the cattle and the land, the land and the cattle. Daddy's friends all said he was mad marrying a 'townie', suggesting Mammy would know nothing about country life. Well, country life was indeed rough but my mammy rose to the task, despite the absence of her husband, who for days at a time travelled to other parts of the country buying cattle.

The homecomings must have been the most wonderful affairs since Daddy and Mammy went on to have six children. There was no contraception in Catholic Ireland, not until the 1970s. Like the very first cat I looked after in the straw bales long ago, Mammy's job was to make a nest for her six children and to keep danger at bay. She needed a helping hand from Sean, from time to time, like the cat needed me, but generally the rearing of the brood was down to Rita.

Their first house in Cappinrush did not have running water and so Mammy walked a half-mile or so there and back to get water from a well, sometimes carrying a child with her. On one occasion, after a particularly obstreperous bullock had escaped, Mam was looking out for it at the same time as fetching buckets of water and, in so doing, tripped over a piece of wood, spilled all of the water just on the threshold, ripped her stockings and grazed her knees, and still had to go back again for the water – because of course there were nappies to be washed and tea to be made.

A couple of years after I was born, we moved to Esker, the home where I grew up, in the parish of Ballyfin, County Laois. I was lucky; I grew up among the cattle and sheep on the farm close to nature and in great innocence. There were no distractions, no bad influences, just the farm and the work. We always had enough to eat and we were looked after. My mammy could make food go a long way, and she had to. On many a dark night, a cattle lorry turned up after midnight with two or three hungry fellows on it and she would bake some bread and make some kind of meal out of nothing to feed them. The loaves and the fishes had nothing on her. No matter how many men were making the hay or the silage, she would always conjure a meal for the masses out of somewhere. She never sent anyone away hungry and along the way she has fed many hundreds who have turned up at her door unannounced.

She could make clothes go a long way, too, and could mend any hole in a sock or shirt in a flash. She turned collars on shirts to make them last longer and knitted all types of garments to keep us warm. This way of life was never to be questioned – it just was. She never expected to attend any social function on time because Sean was always late, such is the way of farming. Sheep don't have special hours when they have lambs; if a cow needs to be milked morning and night then so be it; the grass grows and is cut for hay and silage when the grass says it's ready, not when you are ready. The idea of a normal job with normal working hours never crossed her mind.

The kitchen at Esker was the heart of our home and at its centre was a cooker 'range', an old Rayburn No. 1, with a hot plate for cooking that would burn your fingers off, and a firebox in which turf and wood were burned. On the left side, attached to the cooker, was a tank full of boiling water. This was a massive improvement – hot water in a tank by the cooker and cold water from a tap – so much easier than my mammy having to carry heavy buckets of water from the well down the road.

On the right side of the range was both a roasting oven and a warming oven, one above the other. The warming oven was the most magnificent feature any cooker could ever have. Daddy used it for warming up his freezing feet; Mammy used it for keeping a hypothermic lamb warm while bottle-feeding, sometimes at the same time as cooking bread or a stew in the roasting oven; and I secretly used it one night – which nobody knows until now – for warming up two of the baby kittens from the straw shed. They were weak and looked like they were dying because they were unable to crawl up on the mother cat for a suckle. I kept the cow's milk warm for them overnight in the warming oven too and crept down to check on them before depositing them back in the shed before Daddy got out of bed.

Mammy kept a massive turkey wing tucked on the airing rack directly above the Rayburn cooker, which was used liberally for smacking our legs when we were 'bold' – which in Ireland was very naughty indeed. I usually got smacked if I didn't do something or other right, or I was fighting with my little sister, Josephine, which was often indeed. I got walloped with the turkey wing regularly because I was often 'bold'. Apparently, on one occasion Mam was running round and round the house chasing me with the wing and, giving up, she just came in and sat in the kitchen, while I kept running round and round until I realised there was nobody chasing me.

Mammy taught me to make the best of what I had. She had nothing all of her life and had given half of that away. She also undoubtedly helped to make me who I am, and has supported and believed in me in whatever way she could. She's always been the most resourceful and selfless person I have ever known. Nothing is too much trouble for her. She has looked after everyone all of her life and selflessly given without ever asking for thanks. Her resourcefulness reverberates in every thread of my being. The value of small gestures of kindness is intrinsic to the character of Rita Fitzpatrick. I learned this from the age of seven when I remember climbing to the top of a very long hill to get to the church in Tramore during our annual holiday.

I wasn't the least bit interested in the church, but very interested in the sweet shop next door to it. I can still see it now. There was a machine in the window with sugar dropping down all over the doughnuts that hung on its spindles as they rotated around, glistening in seductive, sweet delight. I was desperate for a doughnut; Mammy was desperate for a drink. We only had enough money for one or the other. She went into the shop, came back out with a brown paper bag, sat beside me on a bench and presented a big doughnut. She broke it in half and, with all of the jam leaking out, gave one half to me and said, 'There you go now, Noel – sure, there's eating and drinking in this!' We both looked out to sea, munched on our confectionery and smiled.

During another summer holiday in Tramore, I was running down the beach joyously brandishing my very first material possession, a multi-coloured beach ball, above my head. I was so excited. I expected to meet new friends and we would have fabulous fun. Then a giant gust of wind whipped the ball from my hands and out to sea in a flash, and my dreams of abundant friendship came to a very abrupt halt. I was on my knees in the sand crying when Mammy came up and put one hand on my shoulder. 'That's a grand thing you've done there now, Noel!' she said. In my head, I was

thinking, 'What's great, what's *grand* about that? I have
no beach ball and no friends.' Then she paused and simply
said, 'Isn't that a lovely thing to do now, Noel – you've given
that ball to a small child in America who needs it much more
than you do.' And so it was – my big multi-coloured beach
ball would float across the Atlantic and some small child on
Staten Island, New York, would be the recipient of a random
act of kindness. I remember thinking for weeks afterwards
that the beach ball had probably punctured and never got to
any child across the ocean at all.

Mammy always made the very best out of every situation,
brought calm to every storm and, in spite of a fairly tough
life, she has borne all of the ups and downs with grace, calm
and humour. Rita has always had – and still has – the very
best sense of humour and the very best smile of anyone I
know. Even now, when she can't move about and is mostly in
her chair or bed because of her disabilities, she is the life and
soul of any gathering, as she has always been, and she can
evoke a smile from even the grumpiest face.

A few years ago, I called her after the doctor had put her
on tablets for her blood pressure. I asked her if everything
was fine with the pills. She said, 'Oh great, great,' and then
added, 'There's just one thing.' That sounded ominous and
I asked what it was. She said that she had been reading the
package insert leaflet for the pills and that it said in there that
she might die. I reassured her that was a standard caveat on
most blood pressure tablets. She hesitated for a moment, and
then with the alacrity of a comedy genius she said, 'Actually
there's something worse on the leaflet.' Now I'm thinking
what can possibly be worse than dying in the eyes of an Irish
Catholic mother? 'It said on there I might get an erection!'

This was all the more humorous because, growing up,

such a word would never have been so much as whispered out loud. There were rules in our childhood and most of them were dictated by the necessities of the farm, or the Church. Certainly swearing wasn't allowed but there were other ramifications too. Rita often emphasised through all of our childhoods that no matter how good one thinks one is, 'Pride always takes a fall.' So in our house, the word 'proud' wasn't much used. Mammy was determined that nothing would 'go to our heads'. I think she just didn't have time to focus on the niceties of praise when we were all younger because she was busy doing what needed to be done. To this day, I still have trouble rejoicing in any success, and rarely say I'm proud of an achievement, whether that be of a TV show, an academic paper, a lecture, or an award. However, I am for sure intensely proud of my team – the extended Fitz-family – who have been by my side as many of my dreams have been realised. They are my big brood of kittens; sometimes they scratch, but I love each one of them just the same.

A cat has a bond with all of her kittens, and though she didn't actually talk of pride until much later in my life, I know that Mammy has always been equally proud of her six children. I had – and still have – a special bond with my mammy that I didn't have with Daddy because I only really worked with him, while I actually *lived* with her. For the five years I was in secondary school, from 1980 to 1985, my three oldest siblings had gone off to find their way in the world, and Grace and Josephine were in boarding school during the week, and came home only at the weekend – so it was just Mammy and Granny Annie and me in the house, mostly alone, except when Daddy came back at night-time. Rita looked after her mother and waited on her hand and foot till her dying day some eighteen years after she had come to live with us. She looked after me too and helped me with my homework, looking up big words for me in a well-thumbed dictionary, which I still have in my office and treasure beyond measure.

She was delighted that I got into veterinary school. Like Daddy, I think that she would have liked me to go into farm animal practice at home in Ireland, though ultimately she just wanted for all of us that we be fulfilled and happy. She has often admitted to me that she has no clue about the world I live in, a world in which I look after dogs, cats or rabbits, because she remains a farmer's wife and in that environment cats still chase mice, dogs still chase sheep and rabbits still run away from what's trying to eat them. It's kind of ironic, really, because as the mammy cat in our house, she looked after everyone. By her own admission she doesn't really understand my goal to give animals the same level of care that we have as humans, because that would never have happened where I grew up.

She had a knee replacement a few years ago. I called her up and she said, 'Noel, you do help all those people to have knee replacements, don't you?' I replied, 'No Mammy, I help all the dogs and cats to have knee replacements, and the technology that we use may inspire new generations of human implant design.' She probed further, asking, 'But you do help people to have the knee replacements, don't you?' I again softly pushed back, but after the fourth time of asking, and recognising that for her and her generation knee replacements in dogs and cats didn't really register highly on the appreciation rankings, I acquiesced and said that indeed I hoped, albeit indirectly, maybe one day to help humans to have better joint replacements by helping animals who really needed them to have them first. Her response to this, from the perspective of a rural Irish farming community, said it all: 'Finally you're good for something!'

It's a sentiment that I've heard echoed by many in the human medical world, in society at large and even in my own profession as people baulk at the thought of advanced surgery and the associated costs in companion animals. For much of society, as for my mother, human medicine and surgery is paramount. Not for me, for that's not my vocation. For me, I love the animals and listen to them all the same, just like I did with the cat and her kittens. It's a beautiful quirk of fate, however, that even though Mammy didn't grow up that way or empathise with companion animals like I do, she still somehow appreciates the journey of love and hope in *The Supervet*, which is apparently on television twice a week in Ireland. She regales me with three-year-old stories like they happened yesterday. Even when she sees the same story a second or third time, she will find something new and fascinating. Strangely, she is intrigued and proud even – though she always uses the word 'blessed' rather than 'proud' – and although she now has a somewhat better idea of what I actually do, she has little tangible understanding of why I do it or of my overall vision and what I aim for with my work.

Mammy is happy knowing that I'm living my life's purpose, even if she doesn't understand it. In recent years when she was no longer able to knit because of her arthritis, she managed to crochet a blanket for me in the colours of Fitzpatrick Referrals. She proudly presented it to me, saying, 'There you go now, the colours of your dog and cat emblem – dark blue, light blue and orange.' I said, 'That's yellow, Mam,' to which she quipped, 'It's orange enough for you, Noel!' Indeed, it is – make the best of what you have. I treasure that blanket and it's wrapped around my knees as I write this chapter, as it often is when I write anything important.

I take special joy in the few occasions when Mammy has got to bask in some reflected glow of any achievements I may have had along the way. When I first made *The Bionic Vet* show for the BBC, it was seen across the globe and I was doing some radio interviews. I had just finished an interview over the phone for an American chat show and there were a number of 'extraordinary' and 'out of this world' superlatives uttered in conjunction with how miraculous the achievement of bionic legs and other inventions were. The hyperbole was dizzying. The very next interview was with a guy from Laois Radio, based in the county in which I grew up. His opening gambit was something along the lines of, 'So, Noel, you've come a long way from having your hand up a cow in Laois.' My sister Frances had made sure that this radio interview was on in the car, as she and Mammy were driving on their annual pilgrimage to Knock, the Marian shrine in the west of Ireland, where Mammy has been a frequent visitor down through the years. Rita didn't know that *her boy* was coming on the radio, and when asked what I missed most about home, I said, 'My mammy's brown bread,' and proceeded to regale the interviewer with tales about her. She said nothing, but furtively lowered the sun visor of the passenger seat, whereupon she started doing her hair in the mirror, eventually asking Frances absentmindedly, 'Do I look all right for this interview?' To this day she has a lively mind and a wicked sense of humour.

My mammy also has the dubious honour of moving the twentieth anniversary of *Riverdance* – a spectacular Irish dancing show first seen on the Eurovision Song Contest in 1994 – six feet to the right. I was invited to go on a popular Irish television show called *The Late Late Show*. This was, and still is to this day, an institution in Irish broadcasting – a must-see on a Friday night that brings families together in front of the TV screen – and I avidly watched it whenever I could as a child. Initially, I asked if there was a mistake as I had no idea that *The Supervet* was watched so widely in Ireland. But sure enough, I was on the show and gratefully accepted, with the proviso that my mammy could come. The lovely lady said no problem, but rang back soon after to say how sorry she was but there was a problem. The wheelchair ramp had been removed for the dancers to line up along the walls of broadcasting house at RTÉ. I promptly responded that I simply couldn't come on the show without my mammy and, as a result, the said wheelchair ramp was reinstated and my mammy moved one hundred dancers to the right by about six feet. Rock'n'roll, Rita!

Maybe there was also a little bit of pride, or rather 'blessing', when University College Dublin presented me with a wonderful award and I gifted it to my mammy in 2014, the penultimate time I have been able to get her out in public, because she is now too frail. She keeps this award in its blue velvet box under the bed, from where it's removed every now and then just to admire it. The other proud possession in her bedroom is the Queen's hat. When I had the good fortune to meet the Queen for the first time in 2015, Rita had not so subtly mentioned on several occasions how much she admired her beautiful hats – Mammy, to be fittingly dressed, has never gone out in public without a hat – so I sought out one of the Queen's favourite milliners, bought a hat and drove it to Ballyfin. It's a beautiful maroon-coloured lace straw dress hat with a bow. I've never seen a bigger smile cross Mammy Rita's face. It's still in its box, nestled in its crepe paper, but is taken out regularly to show visiting admirers, while she beams like the cat who's got the cream.

If I ever have children, and I hope I do, I couldn't wish for a better role model than my mammy. I would look after them and protect them equally and fiercely as she did us six. I would tell them I was proud of them when they deserved praise, and that they could dream as big as they wanted because everything is possible as long as one tries one's best. I would encourage them to make the best of what they have, smile often and look after those around them on life's journey to the best of their ability. I would tell them to love generously and forgive easily as my mammy did, and does. Remembering Mammy's mantra of 'the devil finds work for idle hands', I would encourage them to work hard and fill each day positively and productively.

Thanks, Mammy, for never restricting my dreams and for giving me the freedom to be whoever I wanted to be with unconditional love and unquestioning support.

CHAPTER FIVE

Pirate

My Childhood Friend and the Bullies

When I was about four or five years old, Daddy brought home a new sheepdog puppy. I never thought to ask from where and Daddy isn't around to ask now, so I suppose Pirate, as we named him, came from a farmer somewhere or other as part of one of Daddy's deals. He was an amazing, vivacious bundle of black-and-white fluffy joy that ricocheted around the farm. He learned how to look after the sheep from our older sheepdog, Dingy, and from me he learned about snuggling and secret conversations. His was supposed to be a life of work herding sheep, and Daddy made sure that he understood his place in the world; but secretly he was my confidant, my buddy.

Pirate lived in the cattle shed out the back of our farmhouse. Daddy said he'd never have an animal roaming the farm that didn't earn his keep. The commonly held belief was that a sheepdog would not perform well if not excited to get out in the fields, so from the day he arrived as a puppy Pirate was kept permanently on his chain in the shed, and was only untied, daily, when he was going to work. Having said that, because Daddy was always working, Pirate spent most of his days herding the sheep or driving with him between the various bits of the farm, sitting in the back of the Jeep.

Throughout my childhood, I talked to all the animals on the farm, the cats and the kittens, the calves and the lambs, and the robin in the chestnut tree. The lambs and calves were a lot more vocal than Pirate, while he was a really great listener. I often sneaked into the shed and sat with him, hugging him and just talking to him endlessly. Pirate was my best friend. I told him all of my secrets, and shared all of my fears, hopes and wishes with him. Apart from being slapped at school for no good reason, in my mind, most of the things I talked to Pirate about were dreams and adventures. I'd sit with him alone in the shed, look at my comic books and dream about adventures with my heroes. I didn't know that I had a poor education and I didn't know that I actually knew little of the outside world. These were innocent days. But all of that was about to come to a very abrupt end.

On Monday, 1 September 1980, I was twelve years old and it was my first day at secondary school at Patrician College in Ballyfin. Splendid in my new uniform – grey trousers, shirt and V-necked jumper – I wheeled my bicycle past the ominously imposing Georgian manor house that was once the home of landed gentry and now the living quarters of the Patrician Brothers. Looking up at the big pillars standing sentinel at the doorway and the portico bearing a coat of arms reading 'Vincit Veritas' – truth conquers – I was literally shivering with fear. Amid some jostling and general first-day mayhem of a group of lads, I put the bicycle into the shed to which I was directed, and walked through a large central yard to the classroom block. For the next five years, this daily walk would become an intensely lonely pathway full of boys and noise, none of whom I had much in common with at all. I felt like an alien who had just landed on a different planet. I had come from the secluded cocoon of a farm in a small townland, into a world which I absolutely knew, in every sinew of my body, was going to be a world of suffering – a living hell on earth.

There had been no entry exam or other requirements to gain admittance because the college was required by the Department of Education to have a number of day boys from the surrounding neighbourhood among the boarding students who attended from all over Ireland. To the boys who had come from every major town and city in Ireland – Dublin, Cork, Limerick, Galway – it became clear that I was not one of them; I was a 'culchie', a person from the bogs, which, indeed, I was. It quickly became abundantly apparent to me that after a poor primary school education, I couldn't multiply or subtract very well, I couldn't write very well and I didn't know anything about most of the subjects now on my curriculum. The only other fellow I knew was in class 1A, I was in class 1B, and there were a lot of city boys in class 1B. The other boys immediately sensed that I was different, vulnerable, reclusive, quiet, lost and defenceless. I was a minnow in a pool of sharks who could all read better than me, do maths better than me, knew there were subjects like physics and chemistry and biology, and some of them had even kissed girls – none of which I knew anything at all about! It was incredibly traumatic.

After my first day, I went home and ran to Pirate and sat there in the shed hugging him, crying and crying until I was totally spent. He just nuzzled my face, licked my tears and looked back at me with his big black eyes, in which I found refuge. Pirate was the only creature on earth in whom I felt I could confide. I had no human friend to talk to; my older siblings had fled the nest, and I felt like I couldn't speak to Mammy and Daddy because, like everything else on the farm, one was just supposed to get on with it. I felt ashamed, like it was all my fault. I suppose I could have talked to Mammy and Daddy more, but I didn't know how. There's no blame here, that's just how it was.

That night, my arm around Pirate, I stared into the blackness of night falling in. The thing was, Pirate lived a life of relative solitude, chained in his shed. I felt his need to escape and he felt mine. We were kindred misunderstood souls yearning to run free, but knowing there would always be a chain to hold us down. His was physical, mine was mental, a profound feeling of desperate inferiority that would permeate my life to this day. I didn't know how I was ever going to pull through. I was useless, stupid and dumb, and I sensed that I would never come to anything. Basically, I was screwed and I knew it. We both looked out into the yard with our respective chains around our necks.

I knew, after that first day, I had a straightforward choice: commit myself to studying every waking hour of day and night so that one day I might be able to go to veterinary school, or accept that I really would never come to anything. In truth, there was nothing straightforward about it because many boys quickly recognised that I was a swot, someone to be vilified for studying hard, asking the teachers questions and generally trying not only to catch up, but to surpass all of them in learning.

I didn't know what bullying actually was. What started as giving me 'wedgies' – a cruel and painful activity where underwear is pulled up between the buttocks sharply and tightly – gradually progressed to chucking me in the quarry as a lunchtime ritual. For a very long time, the quarry remained the favoured place of purgatory, as all of the effluent from the farmyard on the Patrician Brothers' estate was dumped here and so I was regularly covered in shite. I remember one time going back into class after a particularly bad and mucky bruising when five boys set on me again, one on each arm, one on each leg, giving me the bumps, throwing me up in the air, while the fifth came down hard with his fists on my stomach as I bounced. When the teacher came into the classroom, they dropped me like a stone on the rostrum. I can still see the look of disdain in the teacher's eyes as he looked down at me and said, '*Nollaig Mac Giolla Phádraig*, stop fooling around and get back to your desk.' I did. I still get flashbacks to that moment whenever I hear the Irish version of my name.

From early on at Ballyfin College, I was called Nollaig, Gaelic for Noel, because that's what Mr Canty, the Latin teacher, called me. I was good at Latin; I liked how it was structured. I always wanted Mr Canty to be proud of me. I never knew that he was, indeed, secretly proud of me until many years later when I heard it second hand. He was different from many other people in that he seemed to understand my sensitive nature, and I suspect that was because he was sensitive too. Many years later, his death by suicide shocked and saddened me greatly – it was a huge loss to mankind. I guess life sometimes gets too much for the sensitive ones. There have been times when it has almost felt too much for me too.

The bullies continued. One crawled into the attic above the classroom and dripped ink through a hole in the ceiling onto my head throughout a lesson. I daren't move; if I did he would just inflict more pain in some other way. One particularly violent day, they hadn't satiated themselves with my lunchtime beating, and when I went to the bike shed to go home, three of them pounced. They ripped my jacket and grabbed my leather bag, sending the contents flying to the ground and, knowing that I'd drop my bike to grab my beloved books, they threw them around like pass-the-parcel. They snatched my bike and careered it down the hill towards a cattle grid – a series of louvered bars like a gate laid flat on its side along a road, the point being that the cattle wouldn't cross because somehow they'd know their feet would get caught. The bullies followed on, shrieking with laughter, and wedged the wheels in between the bars, kicking the bike back and forth until they buckled and broke. I had no bike for a while.

I became somewhat conditioned to the bullying and the beatings, and after I had shown I could withstand the physical abuse, some tried to meddle with my mind and heart instead. It was the mental and emotional stuff that really messed me up, and unfortunately they learned that this kind of torture was easier to inflict, and more devastating. I'd never seen a scary film of any kind, so when they pinned me down on a desk in a classroom, held my eyes open and made me watch Stephen King's *Children of the Corn* on a VHS video that they had stolen, I was traumatised. Eventually, even this kind of bullying didn't work, so they found and unlocked the key to the door of ultimate cruelty for me.

They knew that my textbooks and copybooks were the only material things I really cared about and so they waited and watched. On the day, we were told to leave our school bags in the classroom at lunchtime, so they went back in before me, put a bottle of milk in my bag and perched it on top of the classroom door. They sat, waiting and watching, until I walked in and my bag fell on my head, milk spilling on my precious books, whereupon they rolled around in laughter. I was devastated, totally distraught. I'd spent months meticulously drawing diagrams and writing down the minutest detail in my exercise books. I frantically tried to rescue them from the pool of milk, while desperately fighting to hold back the tears. I was totally crushed and that evening I definitely didn't see the irony of actually crying over spilt milk, as I sat there hugging Pirate's scruffy neck in the dark, rank mustiness of the cattle shed. I cried on many nights during those awful years but on that occasion I felt truly broken. I just did not want or know how to carry on. I closed my eyes to block out the pain, Pirate licking my tear-stained face.

I was still fascinated by superheroes and used my vivid imagination to propel me into a world of endless possibility where neither Pirate nor I had chains holding us back. Now with all of the bullies wearing me down day after day, in the half-light of the cattle shed where I had dreamed that Mr Robin and I would fly off and save the broken animals, I came up with my very own superhero. He would save me from the bullies and he would save all the animals too. He wasn't called The Supervet, as I had no such lofty thoughts at the time; he was called Vetman. Like Batman's search for love and meaning after the loss of his parents, Vetman would bring love and meaning; and like Wolverine's ability to heal himself, Vetman would be able to heal himself and others. I, too, didn't want to feel pain any more. I wanted to become him – he could solve any animal problem, anytime, anyplace, and throughout my early teenage years his story became earthed in fantasy, but evolved into my own personal dream. I suppose Vetman is the distillation of

Batman, Wolverine, the Six Million Dollar Man and Rocky all wrapped up in one. His outfit was mainly blue but could morph like a chameleon into any colour, and his cloak was orange but had loads of fancy features that could become the spines of a porcupine, the tentacles of an octopus or the wings of an eagle.

I imagined that Vetman could talk to animals, without actually using any words – much more accomplished than Doctor Dolittle, whom I'd seen on television. He began to take shape in my head. Having already flown with Mr Robin in my imagination from the chestnut tree, it was no coincidence that Vetman and Robin flew some of their early missions together, just like Batman and Robin. In my story that I made up for Vetman, he was an explorer, like Darwin, out in the jungle looking for new species and new plants from which he could make potions to heal all of the animals like the medicine men of olden times. Then one day in the jungle, he discovered a meteor crater where the brightest star in the Galaxy had fallen – the very same star that I had wished upon the night I lost the lambs. Inside the crater, he discovered magic stardust that had the actual molecular structure of love. Love was in the stars.

I imagined that my superhero would bring this love to the world with what he called his magic bionic dust, and that it would enable him to fix both himself and all of the animals. He fixed up the hedgehog with no legs, the elephant without a trunk, the alligator with no tail, the tortoise without a shell and the parrot with no beak. He took all the animal waifs and strays that nobody else wanted and magically rebuilt them with bits of stuff that people had thrown away – old pieces of cars, wheelbarrows, hairdryers, lighthouse bulbs, aeroplanes and even a spaceship. He also fixed himself with the magic bionic dust and he wrapped his heart in the love dust which he had discovered to protect him from pain. For Vetman, anything was possible.

Vetman had his bullies too, just like me. His biggest foe was called The Man With No Name. He was a monstrous creature, cunning and resourceful, who didn't want love, happy children or happy animals in the world at all. He thrived on misery and pain. I called Vetman's adversary that because I couldn't bear to give any of my own tormentors a name, and I still can't. They don't deserve it; they don't deserve to be remembered. I'd huddle up to Pirate and whisper all of the amazing adventures that Vetman, my hero, had that day in far-flung lands, travelling with his bionic army of animals to fight the bullies. But at school neither Vetman nor Pirate could save me from The Men With No Name who were only too real, and the years of sustained psychological and emotional abuse I endured – day in, day out, unrelenting, unremitting, inexorable and inevitable – have affected me deeply.

Nothing could be done, because it was 'God's will' – or at least, that was what I was led to believe, when I did complain once to a senior Brother. In the end, there was no point in complaining, as it just got worse and 'God's will' was unlikely to change. I am not recounting these tales of woe to condemn the Patrician Brothers, for they were men of their time and, in truth, together with their staff, provided me with an excellent education. Indeed, there are many I could name to whom I am forever grateful. Nor am I criticising Mammy and Daddy because I hid most of it from them. In those days few parents questioned those in authority and, even if they did, there was no guarantee of any improvement – God's will was God's will. I now know that it was the fault of a flawed system that used religion as an excuse for many things. One of those things was to ignore incessant physical and mental violence. There were others, but that's for another day. Thankfully modern Ireland has started to recognise, acknowledge and address these issues.

Looking back at it now, I had a desperate conflict with the religion into which I was born. As an altar boy throughout secondary school, I found the order, safety and certainty of the protocol comforting. The moments of solitude away from the bullies brought me peace. I felt that no one could touch me in my vestments. They were like a protective cloak. Luckily, this was my experience, though I readily acknowledge it was not so for many others. In my vestments, I was respected, thanked and praised; outside of them, the very religion that they stood for was being used as a blanket to cover up my merciless bullying. I learned that a cloak could be used either to raise up goodness or to hide badness. As with all of my superheroes – especially Vetman with his blue suit and magical orange cloak – enabling me to find solace in the turmoil, I was determined that one day I too would dedicate my life, with honour, to goodness.

I tried to hide from the bullies at school as much as I could. I would have gladly stayed in the classroom at lunchtime, but we were forbidden to do so – at least there was less shite to chuck at me there than in the quarry. A few months after the lunchtime quarry chucking began, I found a hiding place that until this day has been my secret – nobody ever knew that I found refuge there. There was an old gardener's cottage way up top of the farmyard out the back of the classrooms. It hadn't been used for years, and had old onions, some shrivelled beets and herbs drying in the corners. The place was full of cobwebs, dust, creaking floorboards and was lit with hazy mist that filtered through the cracks in the wooden door, the gaps in the thatched roof and an old boarded-up window full of woodworm. I found peace, and a place to fly to my secret dreams, there. Escaping after class, I became a very fast runner, and it was no coincidence that I hid a copy of Oscar Wilde's *De Profundis* there, under the floorboards beneath an old wooden bench:

> *Society, as we have constituted it, will have no place*
> *for me, has none to offer; but Nature, whose sweet*
> *rains fall on unjust and just alike, will have clefts*
> *in the rocks where I may hide, and secret valleys in*
> *whose silence I may weep undisturbed. She will hang*
> *the night with stars so that I may walk abroad in the*
> *darkness without stumbling, and send the wind over*
> *my footprints so that none may track me to my hurt:*
> *she will cleanse me in great waters, and with bitter*
> *herbs make me whole.*

I often huddled and listened to the rain falling on the roof, girded by rusty metal and rotting wooden beams. In the winter cold, when the birds had gone to sleep, I lay down among my own bitter herbs scattered on the crumbling wooden floor and felt a little more whole again. I always waited until the distant noise of the boys had faded as they were hauled off to sports or into study, and then scuttled down to the bike shed and headed home. In that cottage, I made friends with a small robin and a nest of swallows who became my companions as I read my school books in the half-light. I liked to think that this robin was perhaps a relative of my Mr Robin in the chestnut tree, another bold little bird bringing the same much-needed message of truth, innocence and hope.

I normally cycled to school, but if he was around, as a special treat some mornings, Daddy would put the bicycle in the back of the Jeep and drive me. However, Daddy was constantly working and wasn't at home much, except at night, and as I always had jobs to do on the farm after school, I would rush home on my bicycle, spend a few minutes with Pirate if he wasn't out in the Jeep with Daddy, and do what was needed to be done on the farm, just like I had done in primary school, but with one big difference: I now had homework and study in abundance. I'd say the rosary with Mammy and Granny, get in turf for the fire, and then go upstairs to sleep for exactly half an hour before eating something and then embarking on a night of homework and study till about 11 p.m., when I'd take a break to check the sheep or do what was needed on the farm again and put Granny to bed with her hot water bottle. She would talk to me while I brushed my teeth and then I would study more until after 1 a.m. and pop in to give Pirate a cuddle, before creeping into my creaky little bed for the night. 'Nighty night, Pirate,' I'd say.

I did this every night during term time for five years, and when the dreaded alarm bell went off, I'd get up at 7.30 a.m. and do it over again. Ballyfin College had school on a Saturday too, so mine was a seven-day week of study, punctuated by work on the farm, going to mass on Friday nights and Sunday mornings, and looking after Granny. I didn't do anything social or have any distractions other than farm work between the ages of twelve and seventeen. This was undoubtedly socially stunting, but ultimately I had to study or there was no hope for me. Study permeated the holidays too, in between farm work, because we'd have term exams, and I was never good enough, never clever enough, never prepared enough in my head. From that very first day entering the classroom until the end of secondary school, I had only one focus: study, and then study more to get enough points in the Leaving Certificate examination. I would suffer the punches, the sneers and the humiliation, because one day I would get out of there. I would realise my dream and go to veterinary school.

At the end of my first year, I was awarded the 'student of the year' prize and received a silver, red, blue, white and golden marble trophy, with a small golden man standing at the top of it. I'd seen Marlon Brando in *On the Waterfront* on TV and it had made just as big an impression on me as *Rocky*. It was also about a boxer, a man called Terry who'd been told to lie down, to take the hits so that the bookies could make money on his opponent. There's a moment in the movie when he looks at Charley, who had made him do it, and he says: *'You don't understand. I coulda' had class. I coulda' been a contender. I coulda' been somebody, instead of a bum, which is what I am, let's face it.'* That's how I felt – like a bum, like a failure – but now, for the first time, I absolutely knew for sure that if I worked hard, if I gave it everything, then maybe, just maybe, I could be a contender. I have a poster from this movie on the wall at my house even now, as I have of many of the movies that have inspired me.

I was of course happy inside that somehow I'd succeeded, that, somehow, against all the odds, I'd studied my way into contention. But when I got home from school that afternoon, I didn't go into the house to show Mammy and Granny the trophy; instead I went to the shed to find Pirate. I was a mess of emotion; on the one hand, I was pleased that I'd proved the bullies wrong, that I was not stupid; on the other, I knew their torture would now only get worse. I wasn't just a swot, I was a swot with an award for being a swot! The other thing that kept going through my head, and still haunts me to this day, was that if I showed someone this success, they might expect me to do it again. What if I couldn't do it? What if I couldn't pull the rabbit out of the hat a second time? I feel this same sense of doubt almost every day, even today. I know I'm only as good as my last surgery. The successes pass by, but I remember every single one of my failures, such is the eternal deck of fortune I choose to hold in my hands. So, I hid the trophy in a brown paper bag in the hay shed lest anyone find it and expect another miracle. I sat beside Pirate and explained everything to him. The lick he gave me told me that he understood perfectly.

I was desperate to become a vet and the obsessive studying became a self-imposed regime – nobody forced me to do it. Throughout my teenage years, I didn't go out at weekends: on Saturday nights, like all other nights, I was fully committed to schoolwork. Studying and learning consumed my entire adolescence, and the same intense resolve still courses through my veins today. It has undoubtedly had emotional consequences for me as an adult, as I have come a cropper in my personal life with this somewhat naive self-imposed credo. The truth, though, is that if you work hard enough you can actually achieve almost everything as long as you stay true to your dream, have a bit of serendipity along the way, your health holds up and you know when to fully commit. I don't recommend a life of isolation to any teenager, but it was the only way for me.

Week in, week out, I had biology, physics or chemistry projects to write up after class, or some maths to figure out. I drew all of the experiments in the most exquisite detail, most of which was entirely irrelevant. I couldn't see the wood for the trees and, if I had, I certainly could have made my life much easier by separating what had to be done from what didn't need be done. I was weak at physics and maths and had zero flair if it didn't bleed. I was attracted to subjects that were tangible and meaningful in my small little life. Numbers were way too abstract for me. However, I needed at least an A or a B in these subjects to get into veterinary school, so I studied them on into the night listening to U2's *The Unforgettable Fire*, which was the only album I had, played on an old black record player with a broken needle. *'One man came in the name of love'* played over and over.

It was Mr Murray's biology class that inspired the surgeon in me. I remember going into my very first lesson with him and I couldn't believe the complexity of it all. I had not seen or learned anything to do with biology in primary school. In fact, I think it was actively frowned upon in case anyone ever asked, 'Where do babies come from?' I marvelled at the miracle that an organism exists at all – I still do. I remember the very first words Mr Murray said to me: 'You don't know very much, do you? But you want to know a lot. I can see that. Good for you.' He was absolutely right and he gave me hope.

Another teacher, Brother Maurice, was my real-life super-hero. He taught me physics, applied maths, chemistry and computer studies. He was the king of invention and had a magnificent workshop of endless creations and curiosities where three-inch floppy discs shared dusty, rusty, oily space with bits of water fountains, old tractor engines, barometers, Bunsen burners and chemicals of eclectic colours in various jars. Brother Maurice's workshop was for me a delicious discovery, where dreams were conceived and realised all in an afternoon. Nothing was beyond reach for Brother Maurice. He encouraged me to dream big.

Mammy, however, was worried about me dreaming so big and studying so much. She came down one Saturday night and said she would 'burn the bloody books' if I didn't go to bed. My mammy is a truly amazing woman and always wanted the very best for us but I was an anomaly – she coped with me as well as she could. I am so very grateful to her for helping me as best she could with my homework and for putting up with me being insular and withdrawn inside my own igloo of seclusion. My older sister Frances also always helped me with some lesson or other, after I'd cornered her on the stairs, no matter how soft her steps were, when she came home from her job as a schoolteacher. When I look at the wonderful things that she has given to her students, things that were never afforded me during my time in primary school, I lament those lost years – but, as I say, it was what it was.

I also have to thank my brother and other sisters for every ounce of help they gave me along the way. John was, and still is, magnificent with his hands, has a clever mind and can build anything, either stationary or mechanical: a house, a car, a tractor. (I often wish I could put up a shelf or a door, but alas, if it doesn't bark or meow or bleed, I'm inept – I'm no good with any tools, other than surgical tools. Though I have to say, I once had to stitch my torn suitcase with suturing forceps and surgical nylon – and that repair has lasted ten years and counting.) Anyways, John has always been an inspiration to me creatively, and if I had half his skill and physical strength I could probably operate on every animal in the world.

Mary has always watched over me like a mother from afar.

She used to look after me as a baby and I know that her love for her special boy has never faded. Grace and Josephine have also helped me throughout life, both then and now. These two had the unfortunate circumstance of being two years older and two years younger than me, and as such they bore the brunt of the farm work I didn't do, because I was locked in my room studying at weekends when they came home from boarding school. I truly am sorry that was the case, but it's probably fair to say that we got equally 'sheeped' every summer – with fencing sheep, corralling sheep, dipping sheep, worming sheep, clipping sheep's hooves, rolling up sheep's wool after shearing, and picking flesh-eating maggots from sheep's fleeces and skin. This was indeed the most miserable 'sheeping' job and involved putting washing powder into a bucket, creating a soapy lather, pouring it onto the sheep and then rubbing the grotty, maggoty, and often deep, bleeding wound like crazy until all of the maggots were washed out. Then we had to rub burned oil drained from the sump of a tractor engine onto the infected area to settle the skin and prevent the flies from laying eggs in the open wound again. It was a thankless, horrendous and vomit-inducing job.

In the end, the long nights of studying paid off, and I won student of the year for four years out of five, and the science award in the final year. That was OK for a culchie, I suppose. I wasn't a gobshite after all. However, the price had been huge – and, truth be told, there was very little that I actually enjoyed about school in those five years. There was one excellent treat, though: I won a European essay competition with a composition about Ireland's place as a new child in the family of the European Economic Community, and went for a week to the Netherlands with children from all over Europe.

I got to meet the Smurfs! More importantly, though, it was the first time I had met children from different countries and learned for sure there was a world outside of Ballyfin, a world that I was absolutely desperate to explore.

In June 1985, I sat my mandatory Leaving Certificate examinations, closely followed by another voluntary examination on all of the same subjects, called Matriculation, which could serve to top up marks. To my knowledge, I was the only one at the school who sat eleven subjects – Maths, Applied Maths, Physics, Chemistry, Biology, Irish, English, French, Geography, Accountancy, and for an added bonus I decided to sit the exam for Home Economics because I couldn't cook, but figured I'd be able to fling some science and maths their way. I got a C! I hated doing exams, and to this day I have a recurring dream that I'm sitting a maths paper in Latin. I had dropped Latin after Intermediate Certificate which was always a regret for me and I believe to Mr Canty also, RIP.

I applied to the only veterinary school in Ireland, University College Dublin, as my first choice. This had been my dream for a decade and I was determined I would succeed. However, in case I didn't get enough points for that I put the Royal College of Surgeons in Ireland as my second choice, thinking that either I'd have to repeat my Leaving Certificate or do a year in medical school and then try to change courses. When I was filling out the application forms, I saw that drama and arts courses were options to study, that they weren't just esoteric and nebulous subjects – neither drama nor art were ever mentioned as career possibilities at Ballyfin College.

While there wasn't any doubt about what I would do with my life, my eyes were opened by emotive poetry and descriptive prose, and I thought I would really like to study literature because I wanted to understand why Oscar Wilde, Dylan Thomas, John Steinbeck or James Joyce could move me to tears. I wanted to understand why words that are written down could adopt a life of their own and conjure up an amazing world that otherwise would never exist, could make me laugh out loud or cry bitterly, and could tap into a part of my soul that I didn't know existed. If I could have, I would have studied veterinary and drama at the same time, but I never voiced this to anyone, ever, as I feared I might be ridiculed for even uttering such a wild notion, and in any case in Ireland at the time this was not possible. It wasn't that anything would ever have got in the way of becoming a vet, but I was determined that one day I would explore this magnificent mystery, however unlikely that seemed.

I didn't know when in August the results would come, nor did I know when the university offers would be made, so life on the farm carried on as normal. The grass and barley still needed cutting, the cattle and sheep still needed herding; the farm didn't care about my results one way or another and I imagine if it could talk it would prefer I just stayed where I was. Pirate probably would have said the same, but, difficult though it was, I knew that like Vetman I needed to fly away. Although it was an anxious wait for my results, on another level I felt like a weight had been lifted off my shoulders, because no matter what happened or what the outcome was, I would not be going back into that class with those bullies.

The letter arrived one morning when I was working with the cattle in the yard out the back of our house. The postman came to our house in the early afternoon and I earnestly watched out for a glimpse of his green van in the laneway. I rarely got post so when one day I saw him drop an official-looking envelope through the post box, I ran inside and there it was – my results – a brown envelope on a brown mat inside the brown front door of our house. I grabbed the envelope and ran off back out to the yard and to Pirate's shed before anyone saw me. I held it in my hands for the longest time with all kinds of doubts running through my mind. What if I wasn't clever enough still? My hands were shaking and Pirate looked up at me expectantly, picking up on my agitation.

Eventually I opened the envelope. I got great grades in nearly all subjects in the Leaving Certificate, but I probably would not have got into vet school on those results alone. However, combined with the results of the Matriculation exam, I knew I had a pretty good shot. I didn't tell anyone because I didn't want them to expect anything, and I didn't want to let anyone down, much like when I had first won student of the year five years earlier.

The university offers were posted on the following week and I got offered both vet school at UCD and medicine at the Royal College of Surgeons. No contest: I was heading for vet school, which was just as well because I doubt that I would have had the patience as a doctor to put up with people complaining all the time. I'd thought about this frequently since I made the application. Pirate never complained!

All I felt when I opened the envelope offering me the place at vet school was great relief. After the bullying and the five years of intense studying, I just couldn't wait to leave that part of my life behind me. I knew there wouldn't be any overt celebration from anyone because that just wasn't the way it was, though Mammy made some of her buns covered with icing to celebrate. We ate them and then it was back out to work. I can't remember anything very much being said; I had done what I needed to do, and life went on.

I have no doubt that both Mammy and Daddy were very happy that I'd realised my dreams, but I think Daddy hoped that I'd come back to the land ultimately. I was well aware that if it was to be, it was up to me. Whatever I had done or was about to do, I would succeed or fail by my own initiative, hard work and tenacity. I never sought the approval of anyone else or yearned for praise or acknowledgement. In that way it wouldn't be disappointing for anyone if I failed, and it wouldn't be so painful for me. I've never expected to be handed anything, I expected to work for it. In a couple of months' time at UCD, work for it I most certainly would. Finally, against all the odds, my dream of becoming a vet was within reach.

Ballyfin College has now been turned into a five-star hotel which has been voted the best in the world, and my garden shed hideaway has disappeared. I know this because I recently returned both to cry and to laugh at the irony of life. The hotel has a whispering room, where the unique architecture transmits sound across the vaulted ceiling so that while one person whispers into one corner, another in the most distant corner can hear each word distinctly. On the day I visited the hotel, there was nobody in the other corner. I spoke to my younger self and wished him well, because it was in that very room, more than thirty years earlier, that nobody had listened to a small, scared boy. I would like to think he heard me, because he's a different fellow now. I wandered to the library where I found multiple copies of the school magazine, *The Tower*. There I was in 1981, spotty-faced and smiling, holding the little silver, red, blue, white and golden student of the year award that I had hidden in the hay shed for a long time, before finally taking it out of the brown paper bag to show to Mammy. I did not look at the pictures of any of The Men With No Names.

When I think back to those evenings spent with Pirate in the cattle shed, whispering secret dreams and flying with Vetman in my head, I often wish I could have been kinder to myself. For a long time, the bullies ruled and kindness had no place in my world. Even today, as I look at the bullies I encounter on social media, I try to summon the essence of Pirate and Vetman. What would they say to the haters? They wouldn't even register the existence of these people 'With No Names'. Pirate would be too busy herding sheep, and Vetman too busy saving the world of animals.

I was away at university in Dublin when Pirate passed away. He was in great health and fifteen years old. Daddy didn't tell me at the time because he probably knew how upset I'd be. He was undoubtedly profoundly upset himself; although he would never have admitted to having a soft spot for Pirate, he surely did, in spite of his functional attitude to animals as a true-blooded farmer. He was obedient and loyal and Daddy spent much more time with Pirate than with any of us children – he was his black-and-white bushy-tailed pal, tongue lolling out as he sat in the back of his Jeep driving around herding sheep. In fact, Pirate was the only animal that I ever knew Daddy was truly attached to on any emotional level. He absolutely knew the 'value' of a good sheepdog, but Pirate was a step above the norm. My Uncle Paul once came to visit and, as was his wont, Daddy asked him to help get in the sheep. It wasn't that a man with one good leg could run very fast, but he could stand in a gap or hold open a gate. Uncle Paul declined and said he was going to the kitchen to help Rita instead because Daddy had boasted that Pirate was as good as two men, so he reasoned that Daddy already had enough help. Daddy didn't say a word; he had respect for the dog.

One day during a very busy season in spring 1986, Daddy was getting in sheep with Pirate and he drove off, forgetting that Pirate hadn't jumped into the back of the Jeep as he usually did. Pirate followed the path down the country roads he had travelled many times – between two of the pieces of land – where we would walk sheep from one bit of the farm to another. The parish church in Ballyfin was between the two. Daddy rarely passed the church without going in to pray. Perhaps more than the cattle and sheep and soil and toil, and maybe even above his family, Sean Fitzpatrick loved his religion. He delivered the reading on the pulpit every Sunday at mass, and was given the nickname of 'The Bishop', which he was called by locals for as long as I can remember. Pirate knew Daddy's routine and went to look for him there, I suppose. All I have been told is that he was outside the church when he was hit by a passing car, and by the time Daddy found him he was dying and shortly afterwards passed away.

Daddy never did give me the details, probably to spare me. I think he blamed himself and it would have been quite painful for him to look at that aspect of his relationship with this particular animal; one wasn't supposed to love an animal when one was a farmer. All I was told is that he didn't suffer. I have said that myself to many people down the years in an effort to give them peace. Truly, I don't know if that was the case or not. All I do know is that Daddy secretly loved

Pirate, and I certainly loved my childhood friend with all of my heart, more than I can actually describe in a few words here. Words are inadequate for all he gave to me during those years.

I miss you desperately every day, Pirate. You taught me the true meaning of unconditional love. I love you so very much. Thank you for listening to me. Nighty night xx.

CHAPTER SIX

A Dog With No Name

Steps to Enlightenment

I was scared senseless walking into the veterinary school of University College Dublin in September 1985. I was seventeen years old, not eighteen until that December. I didn't know what to expect from university, but I did know that I had come from a very insular environment in Ballyfin and all of a sudden I was fending for myself in Dublin. I was beyond naive and rapidly found out that veterinary school wasn't what I thought it would be.

I was living with my sisters Grace and Mary, in a relative's house in St Margarets, which was practically in the middle of the countryside, miles from anywhere on the outer north side of Dublin city. I was cycling sixteen-and-a-half miles to and from lectures each day on a ridiculously thin-wheeled old bicycle with curled-down racing handles, which was all I could afford at the time. The vet school buildings, which have now been redeveloped, were in Ballsbridge, on the south side of the city, and I spent two days a week in Donnybrook on the main UCD campus studying combined lectures with the medical students. On the rare occasion that I managed to get a lift into the city centre with Mary in her blue Renault 4, I was so grateful for a car heater that my toes would curl with pleasure. Ever since those times, I have always valued a car as something one is very lucky to have and how extraordinary it is that it manages to keep out the wind, hail, rain and the snow.

This epic commute in all weathers wasn't exactly conducive to a social life and, to make matters worse, the lectures were far from what I had expected, being theoretical in nature: not a single live animal in sight, only the dead ones in the anatomy dissection theatre. The dissection theatre was in an old Victorian building with pink-tiled walls and white tables, an ominous foreboding place that scared me witless. This wasn't because of the dead animals; I didn't mind that having seen lots of death on the farm. I just couldn't remember the names of any of the nerves, the arteries or the veins that I was dissecting, or many of the parts of their anatomy either, even when I drew them all on my own arms to try to understand and recall. It wasn't until many years later when I figured out what the white stringy things and the red and blue things did that I could remember them. So, obviously, I failed my first anatomy exam. This was not a good start.

Part of the problem for me was that the subjects we studied in first year were quite abstract and didn't appear to have any direct relevance whatsoever to the day-to-day reality of work as a vet. Nowadays the veterinary undergraduate curriculum is much better, with far more hands-on and clinically relevant directed learning from day one, but in 1985 it was learning the old-fashioned way by toiling away to memorise endless hefty tomes of turgid textbooks. I had no distractions but still I had to study really hard to pass exams and, night after night in that house in St Margarets, I pored over *Miller's Anatomy of the Dog* and *Dukes' Physiology of Domestic Animals*. Physiology, biochemistry and anatomy did not come naturally to me, however. I couldn't see the wood for the trees. I created the most exemplary workbooks ever in physiology and biochemistry practical classes, which – I learned many years later – the lecturer kept to show other students the 'gold standard' in work presentation, but I still struggled to articulate what was needed to pass exams.

On the plus side, my daily cycle built strapping thigh muscles and made me the fittest I'd ever been. The one thing I did do apart from studying was take up karate at UCD, in an effort to banish the shadow of my school bullies from my mind, and I did pretty well for a couple of years, kicking and punching things. I was fairly strong and relatively disciplined, and I was finally emerging from my nerdy cocoon. Much as I would have loved to have been, though, I was still no Jean-Claude Van Damme, but in my head, I was Rocky. I conjured *Rocky*'s theme music when I was throwing a hard karate kick or cycling up the steep hill in Finglas on my way home. I even conjured it when studying and willing myself not to give up.

The weather that first winter was brutal – biting winds and driving rain, punctuated with hail, sleet and snow – and so my daily cycle was often treacherous: it was hard to keep a bag of those massive textbooks stable in the small rear basket with the bike's wobbly thin wheels. I remember one bitterly cold morning, when it was snowing so hard, I skidded on a sheet of ice right into the path of an articulated truck, on the Finglas Road, which was then the main route to Belfast. There was no way the truck was stopping and had I slipped three feet further to the right there would have been no study at all thereafter. Thankfully the truck swerved and I lived to walk the rest of the way to the university with my torn trousers and bruised pride.

I couldn't wait to finish my first year in Dublin. It was abominable, but there was one fantastic treat in store for me when the summer term finally came to an end. Liam, who was by now my sister Frances's husband, took me to see Queen play at Slane Castle in County Meath on 5 July 1986. I didn't know what to expect as it was my first ever rock concert. There were more than 80,000 people, many of them a bit drunk, some of them climbing trees, some in dinghies trying to cross the river behind the stage to try to get in illegally. It was the most incredibly crazy thing I'd ever seen. I learned later that part of a wooden barrier at the side of the stage was torn down and security men turned water hoses on people who were trying to get backstage. All I saw was a tall skinny dude in a white tracksuit with red stripes appearing out of a puff of smoke, wearing a crown and singing 'One Vision'. This was a song about sharing a mission, about working together in unison with one heart to find a solution – and it bored into my soul. I could scarcely believe what I was seeing. Under normal circumstances, if this guy, Freddie Mercury, had turned up in any pub in Ireland, he would have been laughed at in those clothes, but standing there in that moment with a crown held high in his hand, he had one of the biggest concert crowds ever in Ireland eating out of the palm of his hand. In that moment, I was reinvigorated and felt that anything was possible.

Mesmerised as I was after Freddie's appearance, I had no mission, or concrete vision, that first summer of university, apart from fulfilling my requirement to see practice so that I could simply get it over and done with. We had to spend a mandatory number of hours in various places over a few so-called 'holiday periods', the least enjoyable of which were on a pig farm and in a meat factory. I got a dispensation from sheep and beef cattle practice because I'd grown up with them and could prove accordingly, but I still had to spend a couple of weeks on a dairy farm milking cows.

The pig farm was the smelliest place in County Laois in the warm summer and, even after showering, I smelled rancid and rank. I had to draw pictures of pig-rearing pens and water-nozzle systems and write essays about pig husbandry, which was so boring, but my worst day ever was when I had to fill in for one of the workers who was off sick. He had a hunchback and mumbled to himself a lot, and I could soon see why: his job was to collect sperm from the boars underneath the artificial sow. It was a mighty unpleasant task which involved hunching down under this wooden beast, into which the unsuspecting boar inserted his corkscrew penis and then the man did what was necessary to collect the sperm in a glass receptacle for artificial insemination. Thankfully I was terrible at it – I made sure of that – and was never asked to fill in again.

The work practice in the meat factory was also unpleasant. A pungent smell mixed with a sickening disinfectant hung in the air. As per the requirements, I signed in, had talks on meat hygiene and disease in cattle, and then went on the meat line alongside a qualified vet to cut lymph nodes in every carcass to check for disease. Sometimes the nodes were swollen or full of pus and then the carcass was condemned. One day, I wasn't wearing my protective chainmail glove properly and I cut through the tendons in my left thumb. Luckily, the sharp knife stopped at the bone. I wrapped up the thumb with some cloth and was off to the hospital to get everything stitched up. Even more luckily, I only have a scar

– but no residual damage. My career as a surgeon could have ended right there. Bad as that was, though, it was even more horrendous to see the cattle slaughtered, particularly when they were stunned rather than shot, then hoisted by their back legs and then had their throats cut. Had I not grown up on a farm, I'm not sure how I would have dealt with that.

My days on the dairy farm were easier, but no less messy, and there the *agricultural* smell was familiar and almost welcome. There was a rotary milking parlour, quite advanced in its day, with a giant rotating circular platform and the milking cubicles arranged around it like spokes on a wheel. The rotations were timed so that, on average – after getting on the moving platform – the cow was milked in the time it took to complete one full rotation, and then she came back off again at the starting point. The four teat cups were attached to a claw with a pulsator regulator and a vacuum tube took the milk away, but the timing of all of this was critical. To be fair, timing wasn't my forte: I was a bit slow, and therefore some cows were not fully milked by the time they got round the circle. At one point I was frantically grappling with two sets of milking teat cups to get them on two cows at the same time when both the beasts shat on me from a height – which is also pretty much how the farmer dealt with me until I learned my milking skills and became a bit more coordinated.

By the end of that summer, I was aching to get back to college. I moved into a house in Stillorgan, south Dublin, which was closer to the vet school. I rented a room from an elderly lady who had one other lodger during the week – a schoolteacher who played loud music in her room. Her music was accompanied by the ear-splitting noise from the guy next door who played his drums all hours of the day and night.

This wasn't conducive to studying, to say the least. To my disappointment, there still wasn't any meaningful learning with live animals apart from the ones I saw on farm visits, and those weren't exactly a novelty since my entire childhood was one extended farm visit. Instead, again there was endless virology, bacteriology, histology, pathology and anatomy to get to grips with. I had charts all over my bedroom wall depicting the names of all of the families of bacteria, viruses and parasites that I could never remember. I had earplugs in to try to mute the surround-sound cacophony as I was trying to learn the myriad of organism subgenres and various parts of liver and kidney cells. The only other thing on my wall at the time was a poster of Rocky Balboa. His rousing soundtrack playing in my head still kept me going through the long nights of study, but not even Rocky urging me on could save me from failing the histopathology exam because I couldn't name all of the bits of the cells. My memory for names showed no sign of improving.

The commute from Stillorgan was less onerous, though, and I happily cycled along listening to Simple Minds, Fleetwood Mac, U2, AC/DC and Billy Idol on my Walkman. This wasn't the best idea, however, because one night, with my parka jacket hood up, I ran into the back of a car. It was lashing rain and I just hadn't bothered to look up. I was thrown up onto the roof of the car and caught my arm in the roof rack, partially dislocating my right shoulder. Fortuitously, it turned out, because I got to sit my exams with a scribe. Those were the easiest exams I ever sat – all I had to do was sit there and think while someone else transcribed: a godsend because my handwriting was – and still is – terrible. Like most people, I write slower than I process mentally, and so when all I had to do was think and verbalise, the answers I gave were noticeably more accurate. This time, I passed with flying colours.

Those first couple of years of veterinary school were very challenging for me. Looking back, I think maybe I thought that I needed to be reclusive in order to succeed, but in some ways I was also conditioned by my upbringing. Coming from a Catholic school, and especially living in a household where my parents were models of sobriety, drinking heavily was something that never appealed to me, and I was also rather oblivious to drug use, so there was no peer pressure of this nature in my university days. The only thing I ever got in trouble with the Garda for was not having a light on my bicycle because my dynamo was broken. There were no laptops, no mobile phones and no internet – social media bombardment and information overload just didn't exist. My generation all learned to imbibe later, but the abstinence during the early years in vet school probably served us well. The Church didn't encourage other illicit activity either – thinking about girls – and so not having to deal with romantic distraction or a broken heart was probably for the best, too. All of that would be enjoyed and suffered later! We had a feared physiology professor who, if one of us was performing poorly, would ask whether such deficiencies were attributable to 'wine, women or song'. None of these was likely in my case.

In 1986, halfway through my second year in vet school, I was still pretty disillusioned and frustrated and desperate to figure out what being a vet was all about. I had even begun to question why I had ever wanted to do it at all. I was walking up to histology class when I saw a poster on the notice board: 'Scholarship to America. Only hard-workers need apply. University of Pennsylvania, Philadelphia.' *Philadelphia* – the home of Rocky! I knew I had to apply, which I duly did, and miraculously I got it. Maybe no one else applied, but I didn't care, I was going to see my hero. Philadelphia, here I come. I was on my way to climb the steps of the Natural History Museum with Rocky.

In a haze of excitement off I went to the travel agent's where a rather befuddled lady was poring over some maps. 'I need a flight to America, please,' I announced excitedly. She removed her spectacles, viewed me with unmasked amusement and asked, 'Any particular part?' With a great big beaming smile, I proclaimed that I needed to get to Philadelphia. 'Oh now, oh now, let's see then – that could be expensive,' she replied. It was. 'Shite!' I couldn't afford to fly to Philadelphia. Seeing my abject dismay she helpfully suggested that Aer Lingus had a special promotional deal to New York. On the map, Philadelphia didn't seem that far from New York – about the same distance as Ballyfin to Dublin – so I told her that that would do me fine, thank you very much.

I landed in JFK airport, without the faintest clue how I was going to get to Philadelphia. I collected my big, bright red rucksack and then wandered around the airport, eyes wide open like the nineteen-year-old gobshite I really was. Eventually, I spotted a bloke dressed in a proper leprechaun outfit carrying a sign that said 'Shamrock Coaches'. My luck was in! Sure enough, Shamrock Coaches had a coach for Philadelphia and off I went. I was sitting beside a middle-aged American lady who struck up banter with me straight away, as did her two friends who were in the seat behind. When we stopped off halfway for a toilet break, they brought me a hotdog and a Coca-Cola. That was the first hotdog I had ever had – and it tasted spicy, hot and most flavoursome, an absolute culinary awakening. These lovely ladies amazingly also paid my bus fare. I couldn't believe my luck; welcome to America!

It was about 1 a.m. when we arrived in Philadelphia and I asked the driver to drop me as close as possible to the veterinary faculty building of the University of Pennsylvania on Spruce Street. The bus drove off leaving me quite alone in this strange new city in the middle of the night, a city street map scrunched in my eager, adventurous hands and a hefty rucksack on my back. I had no idea where I was going. The hot still air was oppressive and I was bombarded by the unfamiliar sights, smells and sounds as I walked a few paces to the corner of the block and tried to get my bearings in the smoky half-light. Huge chalky-dark buildings rose up claustrophobically on either side of the streets and stretched out infinitely in all four directions into the shrouded gloom. I had never been in a city with such tall buildings before. I stood there amazed by the magnitude of it all, looking up and down at the map and trying to make out street names on the dimly lit signs. My rucksack bobbed around on my back as I spun round in wide-eyed bewilderment.

Then drifting out of the shadows of a doorway, a figure was suddenly standing right in my face. All I saw was a black hood, hunched shoulders, a patchy, stubbly beard, deep, dark, eye sockets and the glint of a knife as he brandished it at me.

'Gimme your bag, man!'

He pushed his face right up against mine. I stared at him in silence, totally stunned.

'Gimme your fuckin' bag, man! Gimme your fuckin' bag.'

It didn't really register with me that my rucksack and I were a sitting target on that street corner, and at that point any sane person would have just handed the bag over and run. But I proved a trickier customer than most because I was just incredibly stupid, a gobshite culchie from a bog. Innocent and totally befuddled all at the same time, I said, 'Sure. What would you want my bag for, it's full of socks and underpants – and they wouldn't fit you anyway!'

'Don't fuck with me, man,' he growled in reply. 'Gimme the fuckin' bag or I'll cut it to fuck off ya—'

I learned later that a few months earlier a girl had had her ear cut off for her earrings and a guy had been stabbed for his trainers in this neighbourhood. But at that instant and confronted by the mugger, I knew none of this. Then something extraordinary happened. A black-and-white dog came out of nowhere and sat down by my feet.

'Get the fuck outta here,' the mugger snarled.

The dog, a kind of mastiff cross, didn't budge. He just sat by my feet and started to paw at my leg. 'Get the fuck outta here, mutha-fucker,' but the dog just stayed right where he was. I took a step backwards and slowly lowered my bag to the ground. The mugger, in frustration and anger, tried to push the dog away with his foot; not quite a kick, but not far from it. The dog snarled and refused to move, sitting directly between us – and with wary alertness watched us both.

The man lowered the knife, his yells turning into a kind of muttering of abuse. It wasn't clear whether the abuse was directed at me or the dog or, in fact, at himself, as he became increasingly annoyed with my canine protector, and yet seemed powerless to inflict any violence upon him. It suddenly became clear that it was his dog and he loved him. I opened the rucksack and showed him my selection of T-shirts, underpants and trousers. I turned out my pockets and showed him $250 in cash and $500 in traveller's cheques. Without my signature, the cheques were useless. He was determined and persistent. 'Gimme the fuckin' money, man, and get the fuck outta here.'

The dog jumped up on the side of the bag, which was now lying on the pavement. The guy momentarily lowered the knife to grab the dog by the collar and drag him off. The dog hung on. 'Is that your dog, mister?' I asked, more curious than scared now.

'Go fuck yoursel', man, what's it to you?' A kind of scuffle ensued because the guy clearly didn't want to hurt his dog, and for some unknown reason the dog was protecting me. The mugger was quite unsteady on his legs and once the hood came down I could see that he was also quite old. He wasn't that much of a threat after all. He stumbled in his tussle with the dog and fell over the bag. Inexplicably, I also stooped down and started talking to the dog and to him. He softened a bit and I could hear that he was slurring and mumbling his words when he wasn't shouting them. It was clear he had taken his share, and then some, of drugs and booze.

We just looked at each other for a moment. He got to his feet and I kept talking. I think he must have been worn out by the whole encounter because he just gave up and went and sat down by a barrel in which rubbish was burning. He lit a cigarette, and I sat beside him and he told me a bit about himself and his dog. Circumstance had not been kind to him. He told me that he had been a construction worker with a family once – but it was the sad, age-old story: lost job, lost wife, lost child, followed by alcohol and drugs and eventually the street. He did love that dog – it was the only creature that was by his side, day in, day out, and to a very large extent was the only vestige of love that this man still had in his life. It seemed that he too had found some kind of redemption in his dog. He said that nobody had spoken to him for years like I did that night. I was exhausted but he talked and I listened till the sun came up. As he spoke it occurred to me how anyone's life could turn out badly just through circumstance. My life had been relatively innocent until that point. I had turned up in America without any real plan about how I was going to get to Philadelphia, or in fact what time I'd get there. I naively trusted that I would just cope and get on with whatever happened, which, as it turned out, was exactly what I did.

I gave him $100 and told him I was looking for the vet school – which, it transpired, was just four blocks away. He nodded and said the dog probably recognised I was a vet and he asked me whether I talked to the animals. I said that no, I didn't talk to the animals, I just listened, and sometimes, like tonight, they looked out for me, too. As daylight crept slowly up through the buildings around us, I got up, gave the dog a little rub on the ears, and left them sitting there. The dog sat up and watched me go, the man pulled up his hood and lowered his head. As I walked away, I saw him gently put his hand on the back of his dog's neck to stroke him. A dog with no name had saved me.

As dawn broke, I looked up at the skyscrapers tickling the bellies of the morning clouds, and I felt renewed and alive. Enlightenment and gratitude flooded through me in the first light of that new day. I felt so thankful for that dog with no name, and for lots of other things that I'd previously taken for granted, as I walked along. I had been fortunate, after all, to grow up in a small rural farming community without drugs, without crime and without barrels of flames. I could have been born in a different place with a different set of circumstances, and it may have been much more difficult to see any opportunity at all. That's real life for millions of people around the world every day. I felt very lucky.

Well, lucky until I got to the vet school shortly after dawn. It was already warm, but I had no idea how hot it was going to get in Philadelphia in full summer. The reception at the University of Pennsylvania Small Animal Hospital was open 24 hours a day for night emergencies. I walked in and asked at reception what time the departments would open and resigned myself to wait there for a couple of hours. I sat there sweating before going up to the desk and asking directly for the professor I was supposed to meet. There was no answer on his line. I asked again at eight and then again at nine o'clock. Finally, at about ten o'clock the harsh truth became apparent. The guy who my professor in Dublin had told me to meet was actually on holiday. My early morning euphoria evaporated as I processed this disastrous piece of information, realising that I was in an enormous foreign city, thousands of miles from home, and I didn't know anyone else in all of Philadelphia. My options were limited, to say the least.

To my left big white double doors opened and closed as busy-looking people swiped their cards on a detector. I decided that I could sit there and feel sorry for myself or I could go and try to make some friends. Eventually I decided I'd go for it. The automatic door opened for someone, and I just followed, the *Rocky* theme music reverberating in my head. Here I go; it was now or never.

My bravery soon failed me, however, when two people in white coats came round a corner further down the corridor and headed right towards me. I had been trying to nonchalantly carry the big red rucksack by my side and look as if I knew where I was going, but at that moment I panicked and ducked inside a half-open door, which luckily was a small broom cupboard. I slumped down on the floor in the dark with my rucksack beside me and was suddenly terrified. My dreams of Rocky had come to a shuddering halt.

I changed my clothes in the half-light coming through the door crack, tucked my rucksack into a corner, and ventured out with my heart in my mouth. I plucked up the courage to talk to some people and eventually figured out where to get food, where the toilet was and how to survive for the next three nights in the cupboard. Then two great guys, both called Richard, let me stay at their basement flat nearby for a few nights.

I had never experienced oppressive heat like the summer nights of Philadelphia. Neither I nor the cockroaches slept much. Soon, though, I got hooked up with visitor accommodation at the school and I was finding my feet. It was all so new and exciting: I used my first ever Coke dispensing machine, which seemed a minor miracle in itself. And, finally, I made some friends. The professor, when I eventually met him, turned out to be a really nice fellow and I was working on developing a stereotaxic atlas of the nerve pathways in the brain of a rat as a precursor for a similar atlas of the dog brain. For almost three months, I looked at a hundred or more histological slides of a rat brain and had to construct the nerve pathways in three dimensions, matched to corresponding slices on the MRI scanner. It was tedious and laborious work, but I was looking down the microscope at the future. I was inspired and realised the potential for such progress in real-life veterinary medicine, which I had no idea about until then. These were the very early years of veterinary MRI scanners and, as I pored over the scans, I imagined a future in which I'd have my own scanner and perform brain and spinal surgery.

After a while I asked if I could spend some time in the small animal hospital. The very first day blew my mind. Finally, I was immersed where I wanted to be: right at the coalface of cutting-edge veterinary practice experiencing things that I had never even heard of, let alone seen before. In the radiology department, I met a great man called Jeff Wortman, who, realising that I needed a place to stay, offered a room at his home in return for me mowing the lawn and painting his house, which I was more than willing to do. He explained to me the value of spending time doing things that one is good at – in his case, reading X-ray pictures or scans – and then using that money to pay people to do the jobs one is not as good at or didn't want to do. For some reason, this had not occurred to me before, as on the farm and in school I had just done everything myself. Jeff, his wife Carol and their two daughters were very kind to me.

Soon I met Carol's younger brother, Don Cancelmo, who was just a few years older than me, and I moved into his house in Strafford in the suburbs of Philadelphia. The train from Strafford arrived each morning into the imposing central hall of 30th Street Station and I walked to the veterinary lab with Duran Duran's *Notorious* and Michael Jackson's *Bad* playing at full volume on my Walkman. I also had some copy tapes that I had recorded from Don's record collection – *Brothers in Arms* by Dire Straits, Prince's *Purple Rain* and Bruce Springsteen's *Born in the USA*. I recorded these on a giant boom box that I was very attached to and would subsequently carry home to my flat in Dublin.

Don became one of my lifelong friends, and he introduced me to weekends the likes of which I would never have dared to dream during my two secluded and lonely years in Dublin.

We spent some weekends at a wonderful country house, mucking about on dirt bikes and paddling on a river in canoes, drinking beer and getting crushes on girls, all of which was like a whiff of paradise for me. I got to sit on the back of a Ducati motorbike and ride in a Corvette. I had no idea that life could be like that and all of a sudden my vistas were widened. It really was possible to work hard and play hard and for once I didn't need to feel guilty about not studying twenty-four seven.

Even more paradise was a short trip at the end of that summer to Bermuda at the invitation of Don's parents. That was my first ever foreign beach holiday and it was amazing. Don started dating a girl called Carole that same summer: they married and now have three wonderful children. I had the opportunity to repay his kindness to me when his daughter, Grace, came to spend some time with us at the practice recently. She landed in Gatwick airport, and was whisked to where I was giving a public lecture in London, in front of 1,000 people. It was her birthday so we gave her flowers and I got the whole lecture theatre to sing 'Happy Birthday'. I felt privileged to have the opportunity to repay, in some small way, his great kindness to me.

My life changed forever that summer of 1987. For the very first time I saw what it was like to 'live' a little. I wasn't twenty until December that year and it seems like I crammed all of my teenage years into that one summer when I was nineteen. I saw how people my age were out having fun, and yet I also saw how advanced veterinary medicine was at the University of Pennsylvania vet school. Though I wasn't working in the clinical departments, I visited the small animal hospital often, just as I did the equine hospital at the New Bolton Center. In the small animal surgical department, I saw a hip replacement being performed for the very first time; I saw MRI and CT scans and huge diagnostic laboratories. At the equine centre, I saw gamma scintigraphy, where a radioisotope is injected, goes to areas of inflammation and is picked up by a gamma camera. It's very useful for diagnosis of difficult lameness. They even had a swimming pool with an inflatable life raft to stop horses fracturing their bones when waking up after anaesthesia. My mind was absolutely blown open by all of this. I hadn't seen any of that in Ireland, and I wouldn't for the remainder of my veterinary education.

After my summer in Philadelphia, it was time to return to Dublin for my third year of vet school. As I boarded my bus for New York, this time in broad daylight, on the corner of Spruce Street, I reflected on how far I'd come since first alighting as a naive Irish lad with no clue where I was going or how to get there. In a few short months, I had become a different person, in that I was more confident, more knowledgeable and more passionate about my future direction. I now absolutely knew that almost everything was possible if I wanted to make it so.

Meeting that homeless man and the dog with no name hadn't been the most auspicious of starts, but I realised that dog had taught me the biggest lesson of all. For the dog, colour doesn't matter, reputation doesn't matter, wealth doesn't matter. Dogs see us all as equals. They live in the present and in a world of emotion. They know if you are true and trustworthy, and what they care about most is the love you have in your heart and the kindness you show them.

Animals have saved me many times in my life when I have felt sad, lonely or scared, and this is exactly what that dog did on that night long ago. And I sense that as a society today we are just beginning to realise the value of this unconditional love in a world in which we, as human beings, are becoming increasingly polarised.

If that dog hadn't appeared when he did, who knows what might have happened. The animals I treat are integral family members and many of them teach me something when I have been willing to listen. If I could bottle the love that I see inside my consulting room every day and share it around the world, there is little doubt that we would all be better off, as I was on my very first night in America.

Most people are not born bad, and animals allow us to be the best we can be – I learned this lesson for sure by the barrel of fire. I hadn't found Rocky but I had actually climbed those steps to enlightenment, and I had found a real-life hero – a dog with no name. In stark contrast to the Men With No Name, who had made my life one of abject misery at school, a single dog with no name had offered me redemption. God is Dog backwards, and perhaps, looking backwards, God or Dog really does work in mysterious ways.

CHAPTER SEVEN

Horses for Courses

Hot Water and Hot Tubs in Veterinary School

After a summer of liberation in America, I came back down to earth and to my third year in Dublin with a bang. Suddenly, I was exposed to a whole raft of new challenges, not least to equine medicine and surgery. At that point, I should have recognised that equine practice probably wasn't the career for me. I had upgraded my bicycle to a Honda 125 motorbike so that I could drive to Kildare to see equine practice at a stud farm. Having grown up on a sheep and cattle farm, I knew absolutely nothing about horses, so this was definitely practice for which I needed to get signed off. I drove to the stud at nightfall and stayed up all night waiting for foals to be born so I could learn about delivery. Other times, I arrived early morning at a practice local to the stud to see joint arthroscopy for the very first time. I liked horses, but they didn't seem to like me very much and so I was useless at farriery too; in fact, the only thing I was reasonably good at was comforting the mares before they gave birth.

To make matters worse, my motorbike kept breaking down. One day, I was driving to Kildare and hadn't realised

114

that I'd lost a nut off a bolt in the centre of the frame, and as I coasted along the bolt loosened and fell off, causing the front and back of the bike to break apart. That was the end of the Honda, though miraculously I emerged unscathed. I had by then moved into the scummiest one-room bedsit imaginable, beside a sewer in Ballsbridge. The bed was a wide shelf that was supported by wall brackets and two legs. In the corner, there was a small cooker and two cupboards in which I kept my Weetabix, to which a rat helped itself on regular night-time visits. As I grumpily cut the nibbled edges off the Weetabix biscuits many a morning so that I could have breakfast, I imagined the happy neural pathways in this rat's brain. The motorbike clothing I'd invested in came into its own, however, when I woke up one night and my friend the rat was sitting there, tucking into my Weetabix, brazen as you like. I leapt out of bed and chased it around the tiny room, flinging the door open to shoo it out – all to no avail. I put on my bike gloves and, when I grabbed it, its tail came off in my hands, and the poor rat sprayed blood all over the flat. I finally grabbed it and chucked it out. I felt bad, but what can you do? The rat ate my Weetabix and had covered my flat with blood. At least the gloves saved me from getting bitten, and I wished that I'd had them on the first time I tried to rasp a horse's teeth; the protesting animal nearly chopped off my hand.

I wanted to learn more about horses. I wanted to get better. I was Irish, for goodness sake – and almost everyone knows that Ireland is home to some of the world's best stud farms. I was supposed to know lots about horses. At the vet school, we were finally getting some contact with animals in the yard and one day I was observing the examination of a horse. I asked where one would put in a low four-point nerve block on the front leg of a horse. The precise answer would have been between the deep digital flexor tendon and the suspensory ligament halfway up the length of the cannon bone and distal to the button of the lateral and medial splint bones. The lecturer in question, who was retired from veterinary practice and I suppose may have been cruising towards the end of his career, just waggled the tip of his boot in the general direction of the bottom half of the horse's leg and directed that I should 'shove in some anaesthetic' in that general region and indicated that it would work fine – and then he walked off – leaving me and the guy holding the horse to our own devices.

Third year still wasn't very practical and I'd yet to get near a dog or a cat – one had to wait until fourth and final year for that kind of hands-on clinical practice. So, I started to visit the animal welfare clinic in Charlemont Street whenever I could, where vet John Hardy gave me my first insights into small animal veterinary practice. At that stage, I still didn't know for sure what area of practice I might gravitate towards, but the one thing I was sure of was that I knew very little about anything and had a long way to go. This was highlighted with the deluge of abuse I deservedly got when I used an artery forceps to take a grass seed out of a dog's ear. John told me in no uncertain terms to show more respect for surgical instruments and that they were to be kept for the purpose for which they were intended. A salutary tale one might think, and wise advice, as one should not be abusing one's instruments; but I didn't learn and even now I use all kinds of different instruments for all kinds of different things, leading my interns and residents to frequently remind me I'm not *going by the book*.

I found doing this a challenge, because I was always

thinking of things that weren't in the book yet. The more I learned, the more I yearned to escape the confines of the received practice and found it frustrating that we couldn't be more forward thinking. I couldn't wait to finish third year and, when I did, I was determined to head back to America for the summer. I was desperate, too, to make some money so that I could rent somewhere better in Dublin to finish my studies with the minimum of hassle. I applied for a temporary student working visa and headed back to Philadelphia.

It was my first real chance at a proper paid job. I stayed with Don temporarily and thought maybe I'd go down to Cape May in New Jersey to look for work. I remember the blistering summer sun pumping down like a car engine piston on my little, white Irish head as I walked, still full of wide-eyed awe, from restaurant to diner to enquire after vacancies in my white shirt and my skinny tie. There were gay people, straight people, white, red, yellow, brown and black people, people with Mohicans, people with piercings and people with full-body tattoos: every version of person in the universe. An intriguing prospect. All the kitchens that I looked at were the same, though: scummy. Basically I was going to have to start out washing dishes and clearing tables, like everyone does at the outset. All of that was fine with me – but I needed to make money fast – and in this kind of holiday town, I could see myself spending more than I was going to make.

Don suggested that there might be a job at a hotel local to his house: Guest Quarters Suites Hotel in Valley Forge. On my way in, I passed by a good-looking young bloke getting out of a red Corvette in the carpark. He seemed like he was wearing a waiter's suit so I asked if he worked there and if he could direct me to the banquet manager's office. 'Dude, I own this joint!' he replied, and waved an arm in the general direction. Turned out he did, too – he was THE man on the cocktail floor. What he couldn't make he made up; what he couldn't earn, he cajoled in tips; what he couldn't entertain wasn't worth entertaining and what girl he couldn't chat up, well, there were none. Matt was the all-American hero, and he knew it.

I walked into the office and met the banquet manager, Nanette Hazz, for about three minutes. I will never forget her name or her beauty. I got the job – hallelujah! – and was handed my clocking-in and clocking-out card. All I knew was that I could clock in all day and all night, but the real money was made on tips, because the wage was only a few dollars per hour. It was all about the service, and all about the tips. Being Irish didn't hurt. I learned quickly and the 'oul brogue blarney' was about to come in handy. Over the following three months, I earned more money than I could ever have dreamed of. It probably wasn't that much really – but at the time it seemed like a fortune, and I needed every penny of it to finish vet school.

The only person who knew that I was working several different jobs was the main chef in the kitchen – and he found it hilarious, so we were cool. There was a concert venue nearby and one morning a busload of rather demanding musicians turned up – but it was near noon and breakfast service was well past. They absolutely wanted breakfast – and they absolutely wanted sausages. They weren't taking no for an answer, so the chef – who shall clearly remain nameless – picked all of the sausages that had been left over from breakfast out of the bin, washed them off, heated them up and smiled as he handed the sausage platter to me. They got their sausages and understandably I didn't get tipped.

Clearly the chef wasn't beyond bending the rules quite a bit more than I ever would.

I was making five dollars here, and ten dollars there, it was amazing. I ended up working four different services, all with different aprons – which were hung in a small alcove where room-service orders were prepared. On one occasion, my different shifts came up at the same time. First I was on a banquet function with two tables which I was supposed to be both serving on and clearing; second, I was on the restaurant floor, where I had four tables; third, I was on a crudité reception in the atrium where I was supposed to be clearing glasses, serving drinks and bringing nibbly things like carrot sticks; last, and by no means least, I was on room service. I was changing aprons quicker than nappies on a baby with diarrhoea, and my chef friend just stood there, cracking up laughing. I was frantically folding napkins at the banquet – yes, I did learn how to fold the prettiest napkins – in my nice brown apron when Nanette looked in and nodded that all was well. I nodded back, then tore down the corridor, put on a blueish apron and waltzed out onto the restaurant floor to make some little banter with two of my tables which had just been seated. I ran back into the kitchen and slapped the orders on a metal spike – thinking, right, that will take ten minutes – before running back to the alcove and donning a kind of blackish apron and entering out onto the crudité reception floor where I was a glasses-clearing whirlwind, grabbing a tray of champagne glasses en route and circling around with it until they were all thrust upon most grateful guests. Passing by the elevator door with one glass left on my tray, I handed it to the gentleman getting onto the elevator and he handed me back ten dollars. Result! Back quick as a flash to the alcove where the first room-service orders had come in – through to the kitchen, with our chef friend laughing as I thrust the two orders up on the rail. Back out on the restaurant floor to serve the drinks from the bar, take the food order for tables one and two and the drinks order with some chat for tables three and four which had just arrived. Back to the kitchen, back to the bar, tearing down the corridor pulling on the brown banquet apron, I saw Nanette coming my way around the corner; I ducked into a doorway and she passed by, before I raced back to the room and poured the drinks for the two tables while the guests were mingling. Good, another ten minutes, I thought, and ran back to the alcove.

Room-service orders ready: damn, it was on the fourth floor and as far from the elevator as it could be. I raced the first order up in my horrible green room-service apron – which, by the way, my mum and sister have at home to this day; I even saw my sister wearing it this past Christmas! Back down to the reception in a black apron, more drinks delivered and cleared – I was at this point pouring sweat through my eighties curly mullet, very Patrick Swayze-esque. Then, horror of horrors, a rivulet of sweat trickled down one of my ringlets and, as if in slow motion, I saw it drop into this lady's drink as I served it. Oh my God, for one horrible moment the world stood still.

She looked at me, I looked at her. 'Oh my goodness, I'm so, so sorry, madam,' I said, absolutely mortified. 'You're Irish?' she enquired, arching a mischievous eyebrow. 'Yes,' I answered, as quick as a flash. There was no need to say another word – we were laughing about it in a few seconds, I got her a second glass and she gave me a wink with her long voluptuous false eyelashes, and tipped me five dollars!

I shall remain eternally grateful to Don for putting me

up in his house for another summer, even though this time around I was mostly working. Because I often worked both day and evening shifts, I'd sometimes take a nap in the woods near the hotel. I'd make a little nest of grass among the undergrowth and curl up with a net over me to keep the bugs off and sleep for an hour or so before heading back to work. There was a horse in a field nearby that I befriended, though he probably befriended me because I gave him a carrot or two that I'd take from the bin at work. Still, I'm counting that as one horse that liked me.

I have perfected the art of the nap down the years. I used to be able to sleep anytime, anyplace, anywhere. I've slept in toilets, closets, and any nook or cranny that I could hide away in. I could even fall half-asleep propped up by a wall. I'm still able to nod off to sleep fairly quickly when I need to snatch a few winks nowadays, and I often have to because I think I've spent most of my life in some kind of state of suspended exhaustion. From my very first afternoon naps in secondary school before study, through to naps before study in college, to naps in the car when working around the clock in large animal practice, to naps when holding down several jobs, to naps on the floor when building my referral practice, there have been plenty of stolen naps and lost nights of sleep. This probably hasn't done me any good at all and I know that there are many scientific papers and books written about how awfully I have treated my brain, eyes and body down the years – but hey-ho, different horses for different courses.

Someone else who kept long hours was the pop singer Belinda Carlisle – or at least that was the case when I was on room service one night in the early hours and was called to her room. Of course, I didn't know it was Belinda Carlisle's room until I walked in with a very early breakfast, or a very late dinner – depending on which way you looked at it – because all I can recall is her sitting on the side of her bed in a towel. I had to pinch myself. I had just walked into a hotel room where Belinda Carlisle was sitting in a towel on her bed! My head was spinning faster than a 'Circle in the Sand'! After the initial shock, I was painfully star struck: she was the most beautiful woman I had ever seen in the flesh, even more beautiful than she appeared in her music videos. I nearly fell over myself and spilled everything with fumbling nervousness as I tried to get her food off the tray and onto the table. She just sat there demurely, smiling at my ineptitude. She gave me a generous tip and I smarmed out obsequiously to catch my breath in the corridor.

It was also at Guest Quarters Valley Forge one Friday night that I learned everything I ever needed to know about loneliness – and what I absolutely know to be true to this day. I was on room-service, on a rather quiet Friday night. A Texan businessman regularly stayed at the hotel on a Friday night and it was the same order every time – steak and lobster, champagne with extra glasses – and strawberries with a chocolate dip! Like clockwork, the order came through at 11 p.m.: surf 'n' turf dinner, champagne, extra glasses – but this time no strawberries. Why no strawberries? I wondered. He always orders strawberries. I got the order together and off I went with my little wheelie trolley – but with a large bowl of strawberries carefully tucked away under the tablecloth on the little hidden shelf, just in case. I got to the room and knocked. It was slightly ajar.

'Come right in, sonny!' bellowed a loud Texan voice.

I did as commanded, and walked into the suite. The bedroom and the hot tub were off to the right and I could see various items of clothing – not all men's – strewn on the chairs and, in fact, a particularly bright pair of pink knickers perched precariously on a rather ornate lamp.

'I'll just leave it here then, sir!' I kind of half-whispered, half-shouted towards the hot tub from which billowing mist and tittering laughter was wafting.

'No, no, boy, just bring it on in.'

'Er, all of it, sir?' I murmured, as I gingerly edged towards the hot tub in the alcove.

As I nudged my head round the corner, there he was, up to his man boobs in foam, a cigar in his mouth, with two rather beautiful ladies to either side of him, giggling and splashing suds. I didn't know where to look; it was the most unbelievably sinful vision that this Catholic boy had ever seen. I was destined to go to confession for life!

'Er, the champagne, sir!' I proffered as I handed out the glasses and poured the bubbly, desperately trying to hold my hand still enough to touch the glasses and not something I shouldn't.

'Good boy, good boy.'

'Sir, you forgot the strawberries – would you like some? I brought them anyway,' I exclaimed to cover my embarrassment.

He took the cigar out of his mouth and said, 'Why, yes I would! Yes, I would indeed, boy. Good boy. Good boy!'

'And the chocolate dip, sir?'

Oh yeah, I was on a roll and I was going for gold!

'Good boy. Good boy! I admire your initiative, boy. What d'ya wanna do with your life, boy?'

'Ah, erm, ah. Ah, er, I'm training to be a vet, sir.'

'Eh, eh, a veterinarian. My, oh my – you like horses, boy?'

'Ah, er, er. Yes sir, of course, sir!' Oh Lord, the confession box was beckoning loudly.

'Fetch me my pants boy!'

Ah, now then, it had all been going so well up till then. I'd got the strawberries right, I'd got the chocolate right, I'd not touched anything I shouldn't have, even if I couldn't keep my eyes off the women, and now I landed straight into my own Irish gobshitedness – the Irish gombeen, wet behind the ears. I went to the sofa and retrieved the man's underwear and brought it back to him like an obedient puppy. He laughed out loud.

'You Irish, boy?'

'Yes, sir.'

'Are those pants in Ireland, boy?'

'Yes, sir,' as I held them aloft as though they were a hazardous chemical. I offered them to him, with rapturous giggling recommencing from his companions.

'Trousers, boy! Get me my trousers!' Of course, I didn't know that in America pants equals trousers, not underpants.

'Oh, yes sir, yes sir.'

I returned with the trousers and handed them over. He then took the biggest wodge of notes I have ever seen from his pocket, all hundred-dollar bills wrapped in an elastic band. He took the band off with his massive shovel-like hands and peeled off three hundred-dollar bills and handed them to me, saying, 'I'd like to invest in your future, boy.'

When I hesitated, he insisted, 'Go on, take the money, boy, you've earned it.'

'No, I haven't, sir – I just brought you some strawberries.'

'Listen here, boy. You earned this money because you showed initiative; you earned this money because you used your head.'

And with that he pointed a big sudsy finger towards his own head, having put the cigar back in his mouth.

'Take the money, boy. Don't ever refuse money you earned – you never need to feel bad if ya earned it, boy. Do you think I earned it, boy?'

At this point the girls were sighing and rather bored in the tub while he was having this kind of surreal conversation with me.

'I expect you did. Yes, sir.'

'Damn right, boy. I worked my way up from a farmhand and now this is oil money ya see,' and he shook the wodge of notes at me.

'Do y'all know why I carry such a big pile a' dollars in ma pocket, boy?'

'No sir, I don't.'

'Well, it's partly because I'm partial to a bit a' horse gambling, but it's mainly cos I was attacked once, boy, cos folks who ain't got nothin' want somethin' and folks that have somethin' wanna keep it!'

'Yes, sir.'

'Damn nearly lost ma life – and what good would it all be then, eh?'

'No good, sir.'

'Damn right, damn right. Well, I figure that if I get them muggers comin' at me again, I'll just throw this pile a' cash and it's so heavy that it'll carry, and I'll be long gone by the time they catch it,' and with that he burst out laughing, the moobs bobbing up and down as in raucous cacophony, and he forced the three hundred dollars into my hand.

'Thank you, thank you very much, sir, I appreciate it,' I replied.

The girls got out of the bath – I did the decent thing and looked away as they scuttled, giggling, into the next room. Then, it was as if a momentary silence fell upon the air. The girls seemed to fade away and there was just the sound of the bubbles from the hot tub.

'I know ya do, son, I know y'all appreciate it,' he said, and he paused, as if for dramatic effect, or maybe it was just because he was genuinely moved, I'll never know. Then he said something that will remain with me forever.

He said, 'D'you think I'm happy, boy?'

I just looked at him and said nothing. He carried on after another pause.

'This ain't happiness, boy. Money don't buy happiness – but it sure is a good Band-Aid for the scars – and I got plenty of 'em. On ya go, boy. Don't spend it on the horses!'

Then there was another pause and I turned to go. In that moment he whispered, 'I believe in your future, boy. My future is not your future, boy.'

And with that, the cigar went back in the mouth, the giggling started again, I grabbed my little trolley and was gone. I never saw that man again. There was no order for surf 'n' turf with champagne and strawberries with chocolate dip the next Friday night. There was certainly no fear of me spending it on the horses and I had learned very important lessons which I took into life with me – money doesn't buy happiness, and even when someone seems to be living the high life, they may still be very lonely indeed.

I wasn't really lonely so much as very used to making it on my own by then, but that summer gave me a first taste of what it was to earn proper money. Until that point in vet school, I had scraped by having earned government support in my exams. I'd lived in very cheap accommodation and Daddy also gave me a few pounds if I ever completely ran out. Every pound was accounted for. I wasn't then and have never been motivated by money, but it was clear that it was necessary to fuel any dream. I needed to break free from penury to live somewhere better and so that for the last two years in vet school I could concentrate on study. To this day, I still have nightmares that I'm wandering around Dublin looking for a place to stay. I really don't know why, but I do feel very lucky to have a roof over my head and I constantly remind myself not to take anything for granted.

So, I tried to think of a way that I could continue to make some money while carrying on with studying. After my encounter with all-American bartender hero Matt, I decided that I would try my hand at modelling. How hard could it be? Just taking a few nice pictures and wearing some nice clothes, surely? Well, it wasn't quite that easy. Still, I touted around and finally got a gig with the Ross Tallon modelling agency. I did have a few minor successes and I was the 'beautiful face' of Kilcarra wool on a popular men's knitting pattern the length and breadth of Ireland! However, it became quite onerous walking to the payphone on Baggot Street every day in order to call base to see if there were any jobs, since there was no way for them to contact me. Anyway, there were very few jobs I could actually take because I was busy in class and also, to be successful, one had to *play the game* at social events and parties. I had no intention of playing any game and found a lot of what was going on a bit too hedonistic for me. I was all for having a good time, but my Catholic guilt got the better of me. I did realise that I could get hit on by both men and women. Many years later, I saw that Ross Tallon had become Rebecca De Havilland. I would imagine that in 1980s Dublin being transgender wasn't easy.

On my return from America, I found a nice flat in

Pembroke Road, walking distance from the vet school. The flat had new carpet and no rats, so that was a step up, but it was a few steps down into the basement flat, and was always dark, earning me the nickname *Noel the Mole* from my new friend, Jeanine, who lived in the flat at the very top of the building. Jeanine remains a good friend to this day. I'd come home from college, take a nap, get up and eat and then study into the night. Sometimes I'd eat with Jeanine and her flat-mate, and my classmate Seamus, who she was dating at the time would come round too. Then I'd feel guilty for having wasted time, and would run back to the hole to study. I'd generally work until 3 a.m. before having to get up again at 8 a.m. for class.

Each morning the radio alarm clock woke me up with Ian Dempsey's radio show, often with the puppets Zig and Zag doing a sketch where they would perform different lyrics to popular songs, which I always found hilarious. Then it was time to be out the door. I guess that's just how I have always been built – for late-night action. I am not a morning person.

I was hungry for knowledge and only in extraordinary circumstances did I ever miss lectures. I still carried with me that sense of inadequacy and was as obsessive as I had been since I first went into secondary school. I remember Seamus pushing me out the gates of the school when I had flu as he didn't want to catch it from me sitting next to him. To be fair, I couldn't see or breathe with the gunk pouring from my eyes and nose. I was so attentive to learning that even when the lights went down during radiography film-reading and others were embracing the respite of a snoozy darkened cocoon, I propped up a torch on the desk so that I could still take notes. I was always and remain to this day a compulsive note-taker.

I still hated exams, and the study was awful, but I got through fourth year and after that it was better because we were actually seeing real-life clinical patients regularly, which made all the difference. I downsized the patients I was looking at during the summer break between fourth and final year by taking a scholarship in tiny marine animals at the University of Ghent in Belgium. I wanted to round off the experience and see a few different animal species. Ghent was a million miles away from Philadelphia in every way, and I had a solitary existence, punctuated by doing karate on my own in the children's playground every day. The highlight of my time there was the release of Tim Burton's *Batman* with Michael Keaton. I went five nights in a row!

Final year was intense, though, and I had to work really hard because, as always, things didn't fall easy to me academically, but by then I also had my first girlfriend, Helena, so things were looking up. In the end, I did well enough, attaining a prize for third in the class in veterinary surgery. I even did very well in equine studies! I tried hard subsequently in general practice to befriend more horses, and, in fact, tended to quite a few both in Ireland and in my early years in the UK. I think I became reasonably proficient in equine medicine, and with experience got on well with horses in the end, but ultimately equine practice wasn't for me. The last horse I met before hanging up my stirrups didn't give any impression of what he thought of me, until he kicked me bang in the chest when trying to load him into a horsebox. As I landed in a heap on the yard with two cracked ribs, I figured I'd take my Texan friend's advice and not bet on the goodwill of any more horses.

I still think that Daddy would have liked me to go into

large animal practice and make my home in Ireland, but on the day of graduation none of that was spoken about. No cows, sheep or horses, just Daddy with his lovely suit, Mammy with her lovely dress and me with the most resplendently awful dicky bow ever. There they were, Sean and Rita, visibly proud as punch, standing to either side of me having their picture taken. That was the first time in my life that I knew Daddy was proud, even though he said it only with his eyes. Just like how horses behaved around me, he rarely gave away what he was really thinking. Horses for courses indeed.

CHAPTER EIGHT

Listening to the Animals

Everything Is Impossible Until It Happens

In the end my daddy got his wish, as my first jobs after vet school were at farm animal practices in Ireland. When I graduated from veterinary school in 1990, aged twenty-two, I had no idea what best direction to take. I interviewed for university internships in the UK and in America to learn more in medicine and surgery. It was always the same pattern: I would turn up exhausted from the flight from Dublin and find a quiet toilet in some corner of the university to sleep in, curled around the toilet bowl for a few hours to revive before the interview. Sadly, toilet sleeping didn't seem to revive me enough, as I was unsuccessful in all endeavours to pursue further learning. As it turned out, this was ultimately for the best, as farm animal practice taught me to be resourceful and to make the most out of what I had.

I worked for three vets sequentially during that time – Fintan Graham, near my home in Ballyfin, Paul Rigney in County Offaly and David Smyth in West Cork. They taught me much more than could ever be learned from a book – how to 'sense' what was wrong with the animal. They also taught me that all of the tests in the world cannot replace a good clinical examination. All were farm animal practices and none had an X-ray machine at that time. We certainly had no scanners and we had patchy access to blood tests, partly because of cost and partly because that's just how it was in the early 1990s in vet practice in Ireland. I had my senses – smell, touch, hearing and sight. Sometimes even taste – but that was just on one occasion when unblocking a cow with bloat when I made the regretful mistake of sucking on the stomach tube and got a mouthful of rumen contents! Then there was the sixth sense of knowing how to get 'in tune' with the animal. In general practice back then, veterinary medicine was an art form, I think; not an exact science and certainly not a skill set that can be fully learned from books or cultivated by exams. In the truest sense of the words, this was 'listening to the animals'.

The longest period I spent in farm animal practice was with David Smyth in West Cork and I think it was probably the most formative period of training in my life. I learned how to be an effective clinician, divorced from all of the accoutrements of modern veterinary practice. David absolutely possessed a sixth sense. He could tell the difference between a cow with ketosis, hypomagnesemia tetany or hypocalcaemia, just by the look and smell of her. Some of this rubbed off on me, too. The farmers initially didn't want to see me as I was the new kid on the block, but I'd like to think that gradually I was accepted in my own capacity because of being at ease with the animals, and to some extent sensing what was wrong with them, since that's what farmers do all the time, without any formal training at all. I have my daddy to thank, too, for much of this 'perception' training by apprenticeship.

Nowadays, I often yearn for those times on behalf of my interns and residents. We choose the brightest people who have enormous technical ability as veterinary clinicians, or are particularly skilled in surgery: they jump through academic hoops to pass exams. However, from my own perspective, no exam I have ever taken has replaced learning the craft of 'perception' at the coalface to inform my clinical judgements, before reaching for imaging or blood tests of any kind. Back in the early 1990s, you needed to become *sympatico*, in harmony with the animal because often you were in the middle of a field with a stethoscope in your ears, a thermometer in one hand and palpating with the other, smelling the animal's breath and observing its behaviour. In other words, you really did have to *listen* to the animal to diagnose the problem, because you had to depend upon your wit and senses to be in tune – hearing, touch, smell, sight, even taste – and, yes, faith.

There is probably not a more difficult job in veterinary medicine than being a large animal country practice vet: the demands are enormous and the hours are insanely long, or at least they were back then – which is probably why I never complained about working hard thereafter as a small animal vet. I got soaking wet in the rain going from calving to calving, lambing to lambing, with a never-ending list of calls, taking sleep only when absolutely necessary. Even then I'd be woken by the next calving call, barely an hour after my head had hit the pillow. It was remarkable how little sleep we got, particularly when I was working in West Cork, and David's resilience in the face of this was truly inspiring. Sleep was on an 'as necessary' basis only and work was constant and unrelenting in that vast rural community. It wasn't work actually, it was a way of life. We lived among farmers, like my daddy, for whom work was also a way of life and we were available to them twenty-four hours a day, 365 days a year. Elective jobs like dehorning and paring hooves were often done by the lights of a tractor because we couldn't get around to all of the calls during the day. One night, I fell asleep beside a calf while listening to its chest, only to have the farmer come out at dawn, give me a kick and ridicule my effort with, 'Well, you're not gonna cure him by sleeping on him, boyo!'

Sleep wasn't the only thing in short supply for me in large animal veterinary practice – money was, too. I couldn't afford much of a motoring budget, so when I went on calls for Fintan Graham, who was the vet for the farm where I grew up, I initially drove Daddy's tractor with my tools in a transport box behind. Endearing to the farmers as that may have been, it was very slow and very impractical. I once borrowed Fintan's Peugeot estate and was coming back from calving a cow when I took a corner too fast and crashed into a clay bank. I put a new wing panel onto the car before he got back from holiday – but he knew, of course! Soon afterwards, I bought a fourth-hand yellow Mazda 323, which was my first big material possession and cost £350. It drank more oil than petrol and was unsteady and temperamental; it had no heater and no demister, but it was mine. I loved that car.

Muddy puddles sploshed loudly under the tyres of my crocked old Mazda, as bouncing and jiggling I trundled down the pock-marked gravel lane to the farm of a farmer called Larry. He had made a call via a neighbour, because he didn't have a phone, for me to come see a cow with mastitis. As I arrived at the end of his lane, I saw a black-and-white collie dog limping across the shite-covered yard. I wondered what was going on, but then again I'd seen many a limping dog on an Irish farm, and dogs were rarely a priority among farmers unless they were exceptionally good working dogs. Mastitis in a cow is an infection of the udder, which means no milk, which was indeed a priority. I parked the Mazda by a rickety farmyard gate barely held up with baler twine tied to an electricity pole, and went to find Larry.

He was quite a sight, standing stooped by the half-door of the cottage: filthy, old, cracked Wellington boots covered tattered, dung-coloured, coarsely woven trousers. He was wearing a loosely fitting Irish woollen sweater (a *'geansai'*) with only a few holes in it, and what can only be described as something that used to be an overcoat but was now a kind of waxy tent pulled over his shoulders and tied around his waist with an ancient lace-thin piece of leather strapping. His lanky, patchy hair mingled greasily with his long-bearded face, sunken cheeks and rather bulging eyebrows. His upper incisors, which were of a brownish hue, hung over his lower lip by default because of what I came to recognise as a kind of maxillary prognathism with a bad overbite. It was kind of endearing. His shoulders were permanently stooped, and he wasn't a tall man, so he had to twist his head sideways and upwards at the same time, his neck craned, in order to make eye contact. As a result of some missing premolar teeth, when he did speak, a kind of spittle occasionally spouted forth. For all this, he was bright as a button and had a mischievous twinkle in his eye.

Larry's home was a three-roomed thatched byre on the side of a steep hill surrounded by trees and bushes and a very mucky farmyard with some cattle sheds protecting the cottage from the sweeping winds. He had a few cows but a chosen one lived in his cottage with him as his personal milking cow; it lived in the upper part of the house, which sloped slightly uphill. Larry didn't need to stoop as he led me through the low-beamed rooms, but I did. He was mumbling about the cow's hard teat as we shuffled through the kitchen and the bedroom and into the cow room. The cow's teat was certainly hard, rock hard. I said that there was nothing I could do to save the teat.

He mumbled, 'Ah you're an awful man, you're an awful man, always making problems. Sure, there must be something? Anything?' I had to cut it open with a scalpel blade, as was the norm at the time for end-stage mastitis in one of the four quarters of the udder. I gave the cow an injection and innocently asked why he kept the cow in the upper room of the cottage, rather than putting her in the downhill room, because surely that meant he had to push the shite from the cow down through the end of the bedroom and kitchen – which he did – in a gully that ran the entire length of the cottage. He just crooked his head, stared up at me and said, 'You're an awful man, you're an awful man. Sure isn't she the central heating?' Of course she was. Her body warmth was trapped in the thatch and clay walls like an igloo, albeit a somewhat odoriferous, muck-covered igloo.

Later, as the dog watched us while I handed Larry some further treatment for the cow from the boot of my car, he crooked up his neck and said, 'You'll fix the auld dog while you're here then?' It transpired that the collie had been kicked by one of his cows and had a broken femur. The dog just looked up at both of us quizzically. I said I couldn't possibly fix him right then: I had no equipment with me, it was impossible.

'Ah you're an awful man, you're an awful man, always making problems! Sure, haven't you got all them magic bottles in the boot of your car?' Larry genuinely believed

As a one year old baby with
my sister Mary. She looked
after me like a mother
in my early years.

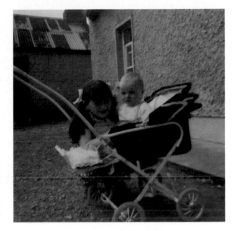

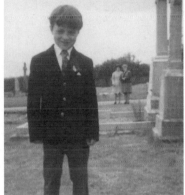

On the day of my First Holy
Communion in my very first
suit, Ballyfin Parish Church,
with my Mammy looking on
approvingly in the background.

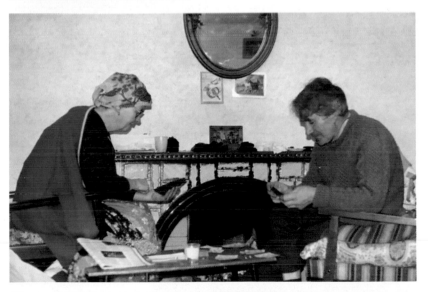

The two most important people in my life. Mammy and Daddy playing cards
in front of the fireplace in our farmhouse, Christmas 1982.

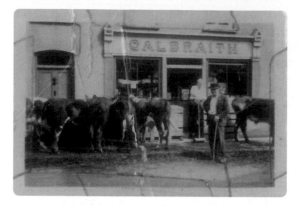

Daddy loved the sheep, the cattle and the land. The fair in Mountrath was his favourite spot to orchestrate the 'sweet deal' (left) and his favourite place in the entire world was The Glebe, where he is seen here herding sheep (below).

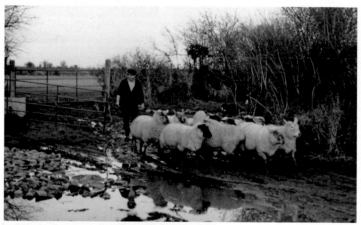

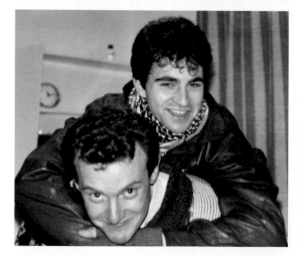

With Seamus, my good friend from university, in 1988. Seamus and I connected over our shared background, growing up on farms in Ireland, and we had many a laugh together through the years.

My resourceful, loving and caring Mammy, in the kitchen of our farmhouse by the Rayburn cooker explaining to my dear friend Rick how she could mend any hole in any sock – she was the queen of making the very best of what she had.

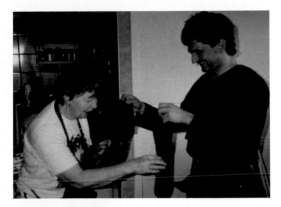

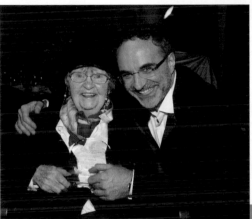

Nobody in the world deserved an award for outstanding contribution more than my Mammy, who I bestowed it upon, having received it at a ceremony in University College Dublin, November 2014. The woman who gave me the freedom and encouragement to follow my dreams.

I'm so thankful that Mammy got to see the opening of Fitzpatrick Referrals Oncology and Soft Tissue Referral Centre in Guildford, September 2015. I just wish that Daddy had been by her side.

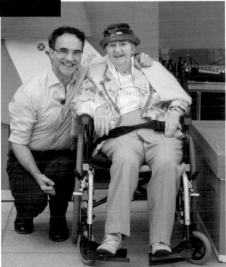

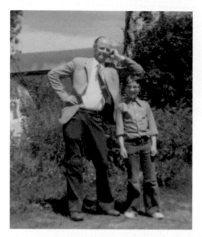

With Uncle Paul, aged ten or eleven. He is leaning on my head, no doubt unloading his wooden leg – the same leg that I knocked over the side of the boat during our fateful fishing trip on the river Shannon. Seeing the pain and distress the ill-fitting socket caused to his stump made me determined that one day I would discover how to fit a bionic leg to both animal and man.

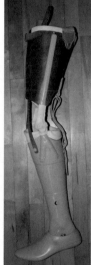

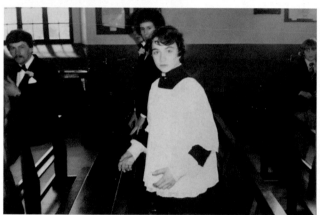

As an altar boy at Liam and Frances' wedding. Liam has fantastic hair and my brother John on the left is sporting a fine moustache.

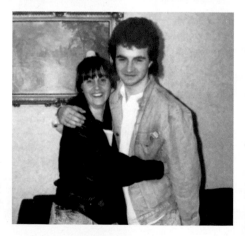

With my older sister Frances in 1984. As a schoolteacher herself, she has immeasurably encouraged, supported, informed and believed in my academic progress and my dreams throughout my life.

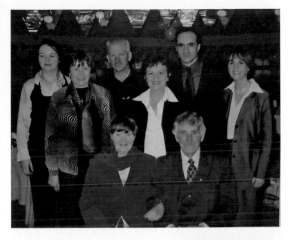

The entire Fitzpatrick family at Mammy and Daddy's 45th wedding anniversary. From left to right, Josephine, Grace, John, Mary, Noel and Frances.

In my childhood bedroom in our farmhouse in Ballyfin, the place where I dreamed of Vetman and spent many long hours studying in order to realise my dream of going to veterinary school.

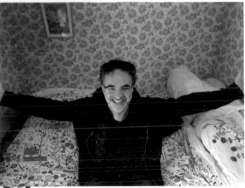

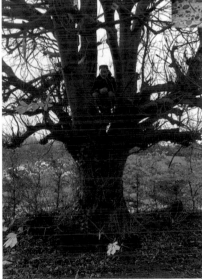

The chestnut tree in the orchard out the back of our house, from where I dreamed that Vetman would fly off with Mr Robin to fix all of the injured and sick animals in the world, with magic bionic dust that had fallen from the stars.

Pursuing my vocation to become a vet – in training to stomach-tube a cow on a farm visit in third year of veterinary school at University College Dublin.

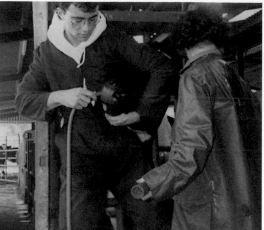

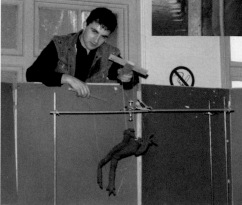

The beginning of One Medicine for me. I didn't want to dissect frogs in order to study theirnervous system, and I didn't see the point in killing more of them every year to do the same experiment over and over again for students, so I made a frog puppet in the anatomy lab and demonstrated each of the nerve reflexes in turn.

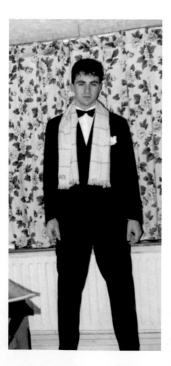

Attempting my best James Bond impression for the graduation ball after finally finishing secondary school, 1985. Sadly, I lacked any 'game' whatsoever in the romance department.

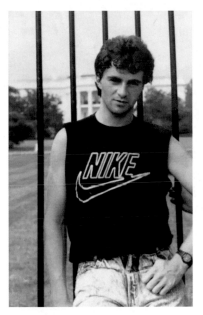

On my scholarship to America in 1987, where my horizons were broadened, at The White House (left) and getting on my soapbox in Philadelphia (below).

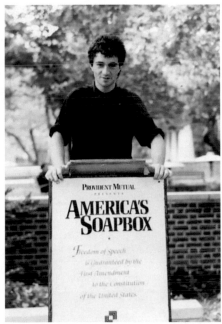

With Rick, my dearest friend for more than 25 years, on my penultimate holiday with him in Brazil 1999 (before our final Hurrah in Australia a year later). After that, building the dream began and holidays ceased to exist.

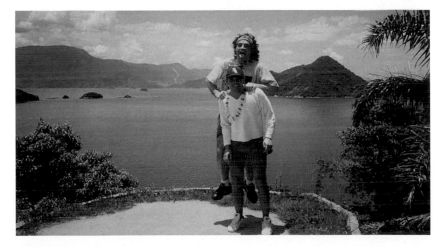

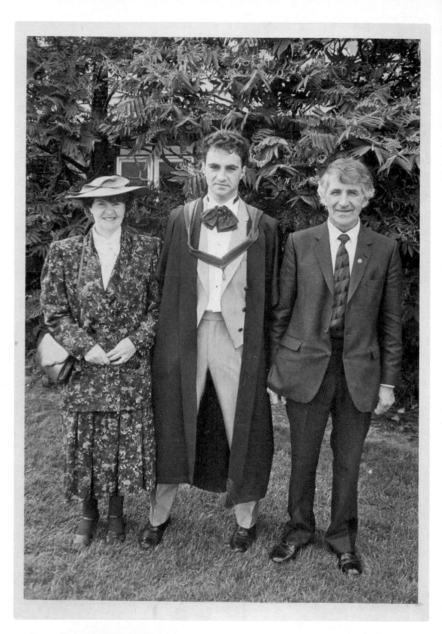

Day of graduation from vet school: Daddy in his lovely suit, Mammy with her lovely dress and me in the most awful dicky bow tie ever created. I love this photo because it was the first time I knew Daddy was proud, even though he only said it with his eyes.

that I could fix anything, as do many people coming to see me today. And, of course, that's not true, but he absolutely believed it was.

Larry lived a simple life. He had no electricity, having stolen all of the electricity supply poles down his lane to build a yard and a shed for the cattle. The only light I could see in the house was a flickering cross inside a yellow glass bulb over the kitchen table – the Sacred Heart of Jesus gas lamp. Moths and flies were committing suicide on that lamp rather than spend one second longer in his cottage. Larry reached down and grabbed the poor dog by the scruff as he beckoned me back into the kitchen. He pushed back the ham and the jam resting on the table, popped a new sheet of newspaper on it and gestured for me to crack on. Carried by his noisy insistence and total belief in my ability, together with the sorry sight of this hapless canine that was visibly in pain, I decided to try my best. I racked my brains and then a second lightbulb came on – inside my head.

I asked him if he had any heavy-duty wire. He nodded with a knowing wink, nudging his nose with the crooked dirt-caked index finger of his right hand. 'I tink I mite hiv some.'

Of course he had wire! He hadn't just stolen all of the electricity poles, but also the wire that was holding them up and as a result had a small mountain of it out the back of the cottage from which I plundered what I needed.

I went out to the Mazda, collected what I required from among the 'magic bottles' in the boot and back in the kitchen I injected the dog with a drug called Small Animal Immobilon – etorphine mixed with methotrimeprazine. This is now outlawed because although it can easily immobilise a dog, it also reduces respiratory and heart rate, and if inadvertently injected into a human, a few drops can kill. The antidote for a human – diprenorphine, branded 'Revivon' – has to be injected immediately, and some vets haven't been that lucky.

I popped the dog up onto the kitchen table, out for the count, with flies falling off the Sacred Heart of Jesus light down around us. Then I shaped a loop from the wire with two long struts coming down from the loop. I had learned this from a lecture by Eric Winstanley at vet school. He knew all about the ways of ancient orthopaedists and, though much of it was antiquated, this top tip served me well here. Fashioned in this way, the wire loop was padded and put up around the groin. Using surgical tape, the bottom part of the leg was stretched straight down onto a U-shape created by the lower upturned ends of the two strut wires. In this way, one would construct a device like a basketball hoop around the groin supported by two pillars, one down the back and one down the front of the leg, with the foot taped to the bottom of the pillars. This would stretch the femur out from the hip to the knee, and immobilise the fragments which would hopefully congeal together with a callus. It would never be anatomically neat, but provided that the callus healing was strong enough and the muscle didn't stick down on it, it might just do the job to provide a functional leg, though often with a residual limp.

This was a Thomas-Schroeder extension splint, first introduced in World War I to keep injured soldiers standing and fighting in the trenches. Between 1916 and 1918, the Thomas splint, as it was then known, reduced the mortality rate associated with fractures of the femur from 80 to 20 per cent. This same splint would now potentially save the leg of this dog on the kitchen table. I stretched the broken back leg out, bandaged and taped it into the frame, and gave the dog a jab of Revivon telling Larry to keep him indoors for a while. He wasn't best pleased about that because the dog lived 'out of doors', but he acquiesced because I warned him that if I came back and there was muck all over the bandage, I'd hold him personally responsible – although that might well happen with the muck inside the cottage anyway.

'Ah you're an awful man, you're an awful man,' he muttered as he pulled the ham and the jam back into the centre of the table. Then he went to the open fire over which stood a metal arm bearing several hooks. From one he removed a great boiling black kettle. 'You'll have a cup of tea before you're on your way now?' he offered. I politely declined, thanking him for his hospitality, and made my exit.

Many years later, I made a similar splint for myself out of some wire, a small kid's toilet seat and an old running shoe, to keep me standing long enough to operate after I had ankle surgery. The surgeon told me to rest up for six weeks, which I didn't exactly comply with because there were too many operations that needed doing. I realise that this makes me a total hypocrite, because I do go mad when patients' families don't follow the rules. I thought I was in control and was keeping it immobilised, just not in horizontal recumbency in a bed. As it turned out, though, the operation didn't work out for a different reason, in that the artificial bone graft dissolved and didn't fill the holes in my talus bone, and I had to have it performed again using bone marrow harvested from my pelvis. To be fair this happened for reasons outside my own or the surgeon's control. So, the second time round, I learned how to carry out my work from a wheelchair, since for me not operating on patients that needed me just wasn't an option.

Do what I say – not what I do!

The next time I saw Larry was one freezing cold February

morning several weeks later on a call-out to cut the horns off his bullocks. This had to be done before the cattle could be sent to market, and was a brutal but necessary process to reduce the risk of injury to people or other cattle, and involved sawing off the horns at their base junction with the skull, including the bit of flesh from which they had grown. I had dehorned many cattle in my youth and I well knew the score. Indeed, Daddy had been engaged in this unpleasant task on the day I came home from hospital one week after my birth. His inability to pick me up at the hospital, however, was not the reason that I have always disliked dehorning. The hassle for both human and animal always seemed so unnecessary to me, since the debudding of calves when very young is so much easier, even though it isn't pretty either, with a burning metal prong taking out the horn bud. Still, no more challenging than lots of the other things that I was doing as a vet on farms in Ireland in the early nineties and people had been doing for hundreds of years before that. But Larry wasn't one for newfangled modern ways – like debudding calves or having electricity, come to that – so dehorning it was on that February morning.

I parked the car and trudged into the yard past the rusty old gate tied to its purloined electricity pole, a tangle of brambles snagging at my trousers and boots. In the half-light of the early morning mist stood twenty-three yearling bullocks, impatiently pawing the glass-thin ice on top of several inches of muck that caked the farmyard. Great greasy tendrils of warm breath and perspiration rose like smoke signals of terror from the bullocks' flared nostrils and steaming flanks. All twenty-three of them slowly turned their heads to eyeball me as I hurdled the gate and landed square up to my calves in the shitty quagmire in front of Larry's cottage.

He was standing at the end of the farm buildings by a rain barrel which collected water from the roof of the thatched cottage. There was no running water inside the dwelling, and his beard dangled into the freezing rainwater at the end of the downpipe from the eaves gutter. As I got closer it became apparent that he was washing a large flat-bladed, wooden-handled saw, the dehorning saw, using a cloth which I identified as a pair of his old long-johns – so I guess he was doing his laundry at the same time as cleaning his tools.

The dehorning saw is a ubiquitous tool of choice for multiple jobs on many an Irish smallholding, and this one was just like one we had on the farm at home that I'd used a few hundred times. Indeed, my dad's dehorning saw is now enshrined in a glass case on the wall of my office where I live and work every day, along with an old injecting syringe and a pair of forceps – the first syringe and forceps I ever used, and the last he ever used.

Across the yard, trundling through the bullocks, I saw two little legs sticking out of the bottom of a rusty upturned barrel, which was slowly making its way across the icy yard. The tiny Wellington boots of a small boy were poised precariously on the pie crust of frozen cow shite, each carefully placed step teasing perilously forwards as he tried to lift one foot out of the muck, and get the next one in front, before it shattered through the thin ice into the murky dung below.

'What's that, Larry?' I hollered, my words steaming out on the brisk morning air, as I gestured at the barrel on legs. He looked up from his labour by twisting his short neck up to the left from his hunched back. Nodding at the slowly moving barrel, he replied, 'Sure, that's the gate!'

'What d'ya mean, that's the gate, Larry?'

'That's the gate – sure, he'll stand at the end of the crush and when them bullocks run up he'll stop 'em'.

I'm thinking, *of course!* Are you friggin' joking me? A small child inside a rain barrel is the gate to stop twenty-three marauding bullocks getting out the end of the cattle crush? Instead, I said something along the lines of, 'But that's impossible, Larry – it's a child in a barrel!' To this day I can remember his shrill laugh of ridicule as he replied, 'You're an awful man, you're an awful man. Sure, that wee fella had a combine harvester drive over him and he was fine!' At which point, I was thinking, sure he did, yeah, sure he did.

Larry said to the boy, 'Johnnie – show the man your legs.'

It turned out Johnnie was the son of a neighbour, a slight lad with a beaming infectious smile and lots of freckles as I remember. He emerged from the barrel, proudly rolled up his trousers and sure enough there were indeed the tyre-shaped bruises on his calves where a combine harvester had actually driven over him. Apparently, the ground was soft enough that his little body sank into it as the tyres rolled over him. Who would have believed it? Larry just laughed and said, 'Ya see, everything is impossible until it happens!'

I had grown up on a farm, so I was well used to the ways of farmers. Their idiosyncrasies held little surprise for me, but this was a new one: a child in a barrel acting as a gate against stampeding bullocks – moreover bullocks that had seen no living creature, other than Larry, for the full eighteen months of their lives to date. I piped up with all of the authority of a farmer's son, 'Now then, Larry, I'm responsible for everyone around the cattle and I just can't let a boy in a rusty rain barrel be a gate at the end of a cattle crush.'

For the unaccustomed, a cattle crush is a long corridor lined with bars and rails or cement walls that farm animals – in this case, cattle – are run down for all manner of things to be done to them, from administering worming medication to pouring on anti-parasitic treatment, to testing for tuberculosis, all of which I witnessed throughout my childhood growing up on the farm. In fact, during my first year in practice I think I broke the local record for most cattle tested for tuberculosis in a day, in the era before numbers were restricted.

As I looked over at it then, I saw that Larry's cattle crush wasn't much better than the barrel in the guise of a gate: it was not constructed of metal bars and posts, or cement walls, but rather of brambles and sticks from hedges woven between more of his nefariously requisitioned electricity poles. To dehorn fully grown bullocks, one has to grab them by the nose with big iron tongs – much like the ones you would use to put coal on a fire. As you might imagine, this is challenging at the best of times, but the unappetising prospect of trying to grab the snout of a marauding bullock in a makeshift chute was looming large as I stomped my foot down and said that no way could Johnnie inside a barrel be 'the gate'.

'Ah, you're an awful man, you're an awful man,' echoed in my ears as I stood at the end of the crush with a chain in my hands. Larry and two helpers, who had arrived, would drive the cattle up the crush. In order to get them into and along the crush, the cattle would need to see that there was some way out at the end. Then, at the last minute, I was going to pull the chain I held in my hand tightly so that a sheet of galvanised iron, hinged on one side, would close and stop the bullocks in their tracks. And so the first one came, stampeding down the crush, head down, the brambles and poles trembling as the ground shook, and the first pair of horns blasted through the galvanised steel in my hands like spears through butter. I can still feel the wrenching of the chain from my hands. In fact, I was lucky it wasn't wrapped round my hands, because I might have put paid to a future career in surgery there and then. (Later in my life, there were several other incidents that may also have ended my career as a surgeon due to my stupidity, but thankfully, so far, I still have the use of my hands and eyes.)

The first bullock pummelled through the enclosure, also made out of brambles and electricity poles, and ran off down the field, with twenty-two others gleefully following. As he rampaged down the hill, he shook the galvanised sheet ferociously like the rusty blades of a helicopter, and in so doing self-amputated one of his horns. Larry gave me a wry smile, 'Ah, you're an awful man, you're an awful man – is that a new technique for chopping off the horns you've got now?'

The cheeky bugger told me I had to stay to help get the bullocks all back in again. I vehemently refused, insisting I had other farm calls to make, which indeed was no lie. Off I went to do some more lambing and calving, while the boys roamed the fields in search of the marauding cattle.

I arrived back at his farm in the afternoon to find Larry sitting by the front gate with his two friends swigging cold tea from a whiskey bottle. In his hand he carried the upturned lid of a biscuit tin, upon which were several Ritz cheese crackers and some squares of cheese. I'm quite sure that the crackers were not supposed to smell of mothballs and the cheese wasn't supposed to have bits of blue and green on it, but then, perhaps mould was deemed appropriate on cheese of a certain vintage. He offered me one of the snacks which I politely declined: it wasn't the vintage for me.

The bullocks were all standing in a clump in the yard,

by now well annoyed at the morning's activities. The gate this time was me on a Massey Ferguson tractor. The first bullock was to run up the crush with the others following him, and as he neared the end and could see a way out, I was to reverse the tractor quickly, thus blocking the exit. Sure enough, in the first bullock went, crashing up the crush as the others followed, with the boys shouting behind them. Head lowered, the bullock hurled itself against the metal of the tractor wheel, and in the process broke off one horn. Blood sprayed everywhere, all over the tractor and over me as I jumped down and tried to nose-tong the beast in order to seal the artery and cut off the other horn. I finally achieved this with the help of one of Larry's friends, only to look up to Larry's usual refrain of, 'You're an awful man, you're an awful man, always making problems. Never mind! That's two down, twenty-one to go!'

With great difficulty in the makeshift crush, each rowdy bullock in turn was held by the nose tongs, the foot of a helper on the neck, while I injected the local anaesthetic and removed its horns ... To everyone's relief, all twenty-three bullocks were finally dehorned just before dark.

I was just gathering my things to leave when Larry's dog came over to inspect the big pile of horns in the yard. He still had a bit of a limp, but seemed happy. Whether he did follow the rules of confinement, I shall never know, because Larry told me he took the splint off himself after a few weeks. He was probably no better at following rules than I was with my own splint. Larry grinned his inimitable smile, and with a knowing twinkle in his eye, crooked his neck up from his hunched stance to look right at me. 'There ya go now, sure,' he said, then repeated, 'everything's impossible until it happens!'

I can still hear Larry's words sometimes even today, nearly three decades later, as I walk into operations that have never been attempted before. Larry, it would seem, was a prophet. Everything is indeed 'impossible until it happens' and I am indeed 'an awful man, always making problems!'

I am always questioning why things are the way they are and how we could do better. Maybe the folks during my initial interviews for internships and residencies felt that I might rock too many boats, ask too many questions or make too many problems, I don't know. In the end, I had to construct my own training programme which would take, as it turned out, another twenty years, in order to become a specialist. This came with its own burden of long hours. It seems like all this time later I still make problems and am still convinced that everything is impossible until it happens.

There is no question that students in vet school still study long hours and this is especially true for those wishing to progress to specialist status. However, I have noticed over the past decade that expectations are changing. Graduates in veterinary medicine today expect fairly regular hours – I have worked with many who simply do not want to work after a certain time, and certainly wouldn't be found de-horning cattle with men like Larry after dark, or working with me on a difficult surgical case after 7 p.m. at night. The profession, in recent years, has become less of a twenty-four hour vocation. I think this is understandable, and maybe even inevitable or desirable, but in my eyes, it's character-building every now and then to put in some long hours as a vet.

Nowadays there are night vets and day vets, sometimes even with entirely different service providers, and that just didn't exist in Ireland when I graduated. Societal expectations have changed, probably for the better, but that's not been the case for me personally because that wasn't how I was brought up, and I have chosen a different path in my career for the last twenty-eight years. It could be argued that a regular schedule actually allows one to be better and more effective at one's job as a vet, but from my own perspective, it was necessary to work long hours for me to make the difference I wanted to make with my vocation in my lifetime.

I genuinely do not expect any graduate ever to work as hard as I do. I don't expect them to work until after midnight, even if I do. This isn't because I specifically want to work late, it's because there are operations that I perform that are quite unique for whatever reason – and there's only so many that I can fit in day or the week. I am definitely trying to reduce this need to operate late, by hopefully training others so we may all equally share the load. I think that a better work–life balance than mine should absolutely be achieved, and I do not recommend my work lifestyle to anyone. However, in one's formative training years, surely one should put in great effort in order to endeavour to be great?

One might think that there are people lining up to learn how to do what I do, like I did with all of my early mentors, but the reality is that it's really difficult to find people who wish to take on the risk profile of advanced surgical interventions and the inevitable stress that comes with that choice. Junior trainees and senior specialists can get easier positions. I often worry about how I might inspire future generations to realise that striving for greatness is worth it, as is learning by listening to the animals in an apprenticeship of purpose, however long that takes, rather than just cramming from a textbook to pass an examination.

I think it would be wonderful if we could select veterinary undergraduates on the breadth of the senses in their grasp, and the scope of compassion in their hearts or their vehement determination to work as hard as is necessary to become great, but sadly these things can't be measured. So we choose people purely on the basis of their exposure to animals and their skill in passing exams. We can't measure compassion, clinical acumen or dedication easily in written exams, and even in one-to-one interviews it's very difficult and very subjective. Furthermore, in the modern era of legalities, students can claim unfair treatment if the criterion for marking is not tangible and objective, without any adjudication of subjective qualities.

Yet, from my experience over the years I've learned that while guardians of an animal want their vet to be the most brilliant clinical scientist, they also want them to *care* desperately. *'People don't care what you know until they know that you care.'* I often say this to interns and residents. I think all of these factors need to be taken into consideration as curricula evolve, especially as students today choose very early on in their education which 'elective' studies they wish to pursue. Vet schools try to educate every student so that they have an understanding of how to treat all species of animals, but this is increasingly difficult as the demands of farm animal practice, equine practice, and companion animal practice – not to mention wild species and zoo animal practice – are so wildly disparate.

Imagine asking students of human medicine to study several different species in their undergraduate career. To make this even more of a challenge, like human medicine, veterinary medicine is becoming super-specialised. Today I mostly perform surgery using custom implants and advanced salvage techniques. In human surgery there are clinicians who specialise in only wrist surgery or ankle surgery, or only perform revision surgeries, or only operate on the retina of the eyeball. Yet clients still expect to be able to turn to their local vet to mend a fracture, or to open an abdomen and take out a spleen. I personally feel that increasingly this will no longer be the case in veterinary medicine, in the near future, as society grows more aware of the options and as young vets make different choices.

Farming has also changed beyond recognition since I was first in practice. Many of the smallholdings that we served back then would no longer be viable in the modern and more intensified agricultural era. I doubt that there are many farmers like Larry left nowadays. Another reality for vets at that time was that many farmers, including my own father, rarely paid the vet directly after treatment of an animal. Often they'd say that they'd pay after harvest, or after calving season, or whatever, and eventually when they came to settle their accounts they would try to get money off the bill. In this way many vets lived in a world of financial uncertainty, having worked all winter and spring and gone on numerous calls to a farm, and ending up having to give discounts for work already done. This has changed considerably and much of veterinary medicine and agriculture has been monetised beyond recognition. This is also shaping the expectations of the modern graduate – which is understandable, of course, as they have spent considerable financial resource on their education. Nevertheless, they do expect and undoubtedly deserve a good wage, regular hours and a nice place to stay from day one. I don't think that the likes of Larry and his dog on the kitchen table will ever be seen again in our part of the world. I yearn to give veterinary graduates a sense of what this kind of improvisation and thought process felt like, but alas, I fear the time has passed.

When I started out, I couldn't afford much of a place to stay at, so in the early days, I lived in some less than salubrious surroundings. The worst was one of two flats above a public house and a funeral parlour. Needless to say, with a corpse frequently laid out below, the place was constantly freezing. The landlord owned all three – flats, pub and funeral parlour – the master of life and death in that town. While you were alive, and could drink enough to mourn the dead, he was making money; and when you were dead your money still ended up in his pocket. He was tight with the shillings and the two flats were actually one room split in two, but being too miserly to buy two baths or two showers, he had simply built a wall through an old metal bath, drilled a plughole in the non-plughole end, and erected a shower head on each side of the wall above the half-bath, with mastic sealant along the wall edges, thus providing a shower for each half of the flat. The guy who lived in the other flat worked in the pub and when he came in at closing time, which was generally about 1 a.m., and took a shower, the water dribbled through the sealant to my side of the bath. Ah, those were the days!

The bottom of my Mazda was also leaky with rust and I had shored it up with sealant. This worked for a while until one night when I was coming back from doing a caesarean on a cow in the early hours. It was raining and the windscreen wipers were broken, the demister didn't work and, with the aid of a newspaper to wipe the inside of the screen, and driving at a certain speed to meet the rain, I could just about see where I was going. I was knackered and grumpy and got a puncture. Of course, I had to haul all of the kit out of the boot of the car to get the spare wheel. I changed the wheel, put the kit back in and drove off, only to realise when I got near home that I'd left the punctured wheel on the side of the road. I was well and truly seething as I drove back, located the wheel in the dark and lashing rain and banged it into the boot on top of everything.

I didn't realise until the following morning that I had thrown the wheel in with such force that the rusty bottom of the boot had fallen out. All of my bottles of medicine and surgery kit had fallen out along the road and all that was left was a calving jack wedged in the gaping hole, with the punctured wheel balanced on top of it. The car was so noisy anyway and it was raining so hard that I had been focused on driving and not on the noise of my kit falling out bit by bit over several miles of country road. I had to retrace my route all the way, find and pick up what I could and bemoan the loss of many bottles of antibiotics, magnesium, calcium and various other vital accoutrements of my trade.

I didn't fare any better when I swapped the Mazda for my very first new car – a Peugeot 206. I was again coming home from calving a cow one night, in a blanket of fog along a very windy country lane, of which there were many in West Cork. I was driving too fast and suddenly saw a wall in front of me. It was the wall of a bridge turning to my left, so to avoid it I swerved right and drove straight into the river. My descent was broken by a tree stump and, as the car came to an abrupt stop, a large bottle of euthanasia solution flew off one of the shelves in the back of the car and smashed on the back of my head – the shelves were makeshift, hammered together from some old planks of wood. I was very lucky I wasn't killed by driving further into the river, by the collision with the tree stump or by the big gash in the back of my head that was splattered with Euthatal. I was gutted that my new car was toast. I could only hope to become a better vet than I was a driver.

My years in country practice were character-building: the places I lived, the farmers I met, the cars I drove, the animals I got to listen to, the experience I gleaned. All of it has served me well in later life. I think that I possibly would have made a good farm animal vet if I'd stuck at it. I could have had a different life, maybe living on the side of a hill somewhere with kids and a farm of our own. I wouldn't have lived with my milking cow in the spare room, but each to his own!

However, that life wasn't for me. I grew frustrated that I couldn't push things further. I was hungry for more and, having been to America, I'd already had a flavour of what was possible in the veterinary world. I knew there was much more out there that could possibly be achieved. I had seen brilliant surgeons at work and I had seen a new era of diagnostic imaging and implants beginning to emerge. I wondered why veterinary medics didn't embrace change like our human medical colleagues. I could have had a very different life if I'd chosen human medicine when I was offered a place at the Royal College of Surgeons in Dublin all those years earlier, but animals and their well-being was my calling then, is my calling now, and will remain my vocation until the end.

I knew that all human medicine needed an animal model, and I had an idea that somehow I could make veterinary medicine better and maybe have a role in helping human medicine, too. This premise has become the central core of my life endeavour. For a couple of hundred years, humans have experimentally given a disease to an animal to test a drug or an implant for human benefit. I question why it is so difficult to make new drugs and implants available to treat animals where that disease or disability is naturally occurring, but of course only where other options are at best sub-optimal, or sometimes non-existent and within an appropriate ethical framework. This may help the animal better than the status quo, and might also be a superior model from which human medics can learn too, whether it's cancer or arthritis for example, provided that all reasonable argument and legal governance dictates that it's likely better than what we can offer otherwise. Of course this is simplistic, but the basic premise is that in saving the life or limb of that animal, one can save the life or limb of a human without the need to take the life of an animal. This is One Medicine, and back at the beginning it really did seem like an impossible dream. I am determined in my lifetime to bring this concept to the very core of public consciousness, and to give animals a fair deal as we move both veterinary and human medicine forward. In this continuing struggle today to change the status quo, I'm quite sure that I have been seen by many as 'always making problems'.

Another impossible dream still nestling in my young soul at that time was that of studying arts as well as science. I could not get it out of my head, or my heart, that the joy and escape I experienced in a book, or a play, or a film, was not somehow part of the rich tapestry I could weave into my life to enhance it and something I could use to translate this vision of medicine to the wider world. I had found refuge in Wolverine and Vetman as a child, in Dylan Thomas and Oscar Wilde as an adolescent and in films like *The Mission* as a young adult. I remember sitting in the cinema after my exams in 1987 and watching that film three times in one day and crying each and every time. I just stayed in the cinema all day for all three showings – nobody bothered me. Somehow I could empathise with complete and absolute faith in a mission.

In spite of the odds against it, in my naive innocence, I dreamed that this mission was possible: to positively change the future of veterinary and human medicine in a tangible and lasting way, and to figure out how to communicate this to the world. It was a crazy idea, but I knew I only had one life, and I was determined to make an impact. Then it happened, my blinding explosion of epiphany – a literal impact – from the arse of a cow: diarrhoea on my head, over my ears and in my eyes.

I was paring the cow's hooves by the lights of a Massey Ferguson tractor late into the evening because I'd been busy all day with calving and lambing. The cow's back hoof was nestled on the plastic leggings of my knee as I pared off her ingrown claw and removed the nasty abscess in there. My arse was perched up against her buttocks, when I hit a sensitive bit. In response, she let loose with the biggest deluge of watery shit all over my head. In that moment, as I stood up and wiped the excrement from my hair, eyes and ears, I thought to myself: my time here is done.

The goal of becoming a specialist in America wasn't going to happen as I had been refused every interview, so I determined that I would go to England. I chose London because I was chasing the dream of becoming a specialist and studying drama too. There were plenty of veterinary jobs for those prepared to work hard, and I was no stranger to that.

Soon afterwards, I was in Heathrow airport with the headphones of my Walkman in my ears. I was listening to Take That. I knew it wasn't likely that my aspirations would 'only take a minute'. I was in it for the long haul. I couldn't end up further back than where I'd started. It was also highly likely that I would 'never forget' where I was coming from, because I had no money, no prospects and very little experience of working with companion animals. I did have a head full of dreams and a heart full of good intentions, though, as I set out with Larry's words echoing in my mind. 'Everything's impossible until it happens!'

CHAPTER NINE

Carving Out My Way

A Foot in Both Camps

A car drew up and parked hastily on the pavement outside the surgery shopfront on a residential street in Guildford, Surrey, at my first job in the UK. A man, dressed in carpenter's overalls, jumped out and carried his hairy black-and-white crossbreed into the waiting room. The dog's back leg was hanging limp over the arm of the man who was in a right state. The dog, however, was remarkably calm, as if he'd put up with anything. Later, I learned that he was a rescue dog who'd been saved from a difficult situation.

I took the dog into the examination room and did my best to calm the man down. His carpenter's table had fallen on the dog's leg and broken his shin bone. Fortunately it wasn't as bad as it looked and I sedated the dog and sent the man on his way. I reckoned that no major intervention was required, which was just as well, because at that stage of my career, I wasn't experienced enough for major interventions. The broken tibia would probably be fine with just a plaster cast. When the guy came to pick him up, he'd carved a little wooden dog for me to say thanks.

It turned out that the dog had rescued this man, too; he'd had a rough time with alcohol, among other things, after his wife left him. His dog did fine and, to my knowledge, he did too. Time and time again, throughout my career, and in my own life, I have seen how animals pick people up when they have fallen or when their relationships have failed. I saved that little wooden canine as a good luck charm in carving out my path.

After arriving in the UK, I registered with the Royal College of Veterinary Surgeons on 3 July 1991 and signed up with a locum agency to do temporary work. My first job was in Guildford at a small animal practice run by a vet called Michael Alder. I didn't interview: Michael needed a locum, the agency sent me, so I turned up one Monday morning. Guildford was near London, and that was where I figured I could chase my dreams of becoming the best vet I could be and possibly attend drama school there, too. Guildford was a culture shock: it was most definitely a different environment from West Cork and I knew not a soul, but I knew that I'd have to endure some fear and loneliness if I wanted to progress.

Mike and his wife, Diane, were patient and kind and looked after me very well, putting me up in their house and then in a flat above their practice. Mike and his nurses taught me more about practical matters in a small animal veterinary practice in a few months than I had learned in the entirety of vet school, and I'm forever grateful. I strongly believed then, and still do today, that veterinary nurses are the lifeblood of companion animal veterinary practice and I know that I am indebted to all those who have taught me, supported me and stood by my side in countless challenging circumstances down the years. From them, I have learned how to be strong in the face of adversity and, to a large extent, they have propelled me to think big and strive for finding better ways of doing things in veterinary medicine.

Eventually, I became quite good at routine soft-tissue surgery and even saw Mike perform some orthopaedics. The contrast between general practice in Ireland and small animal practice in the UK was illuminating and I gleaned knowledge wherever I could. I was enjoying work in Guildford, but I kept a foot in both camps as I had promised to return to West Cork for a long spring to help David Smyth with more lambing and calving. My plan was to work in the UK for the rest of 1991, spend spring 1992 in Ireland and then come back to Guildford.

Dividing my time between Guildford and Ireland during this period, it became clear to me that, in the UK at least, the days of mixed practice, working as a vet who treated both small and large animals, were numbered, because the demands faced by vets for dogs and cats were so vastly different to those faced by vets for cows and sheep. By the early nineties, the veterinary profession in the UK was diverging, and equine practice, too, was becoming more specific: performance horse clients demanded a higher level of care than that which could be offered through a general practitioner's skill set.

I had been accustomed to an environment where the local vet was the port of call for all species and, when treatment wasn't possible, the animal was simply put to sleep. There was a rather utilitarian attitude to animals in the farming community, as there had been for my daddy when I was growing up – and even in the Charlemont Street small animal hospital, where I had seen practice in Dublin, or in the small animal hospital in UCD, most clients didn't have enough money for specialist treatment and surgery, or did not wish to spend the money because the life of a dog or a cat was appreciated differently.

The value placed on the life of a dog or a cat varies in every country and every circumstance, but when animals are integral to a family, they can tell us more about ourselves than we might care to admit. I have seen relationships become closer or fall apart in my consulting room over the crisis of a dog or cat, and over arguments about money. I have also been to weddings that were consolidated in my consulting room and seen longstanding couples grow closer when they make life-or-death decisions over the treatment of their animal friend.

Alas, not so on one occasion when I was working in another small animal practice. One afternoon, between consultations, I stood and watched from the consulting room window as a gorgeous Bentley drove into the yard. A beautiful lady, impeccably dressed and manicured, emerged from the passenger seat clutching a Louis Vuitton handbag. A suited gentleman, who I took to be her husband, followed. He was carrying a small West Highland terrier, seemingly in some distress, so I went out to greet them as they came into reception and ushered them through to my room. I could now see that the poor dog was vomiting and was clearly trying to bring something up, so I asked if he might have swallowed anything. The couple shrugged and said they didn't know.

I clinically examined the terrier and felt it best to administer some emetic apomorphine to try to make him vomit everything up before doing anything more invasive. We all went out onto a patch of grass in front of the practice to let him sniff around for a bit and hopefully bring up whatever was causing him to retch. We hadn't long to wait. Heave, heave, heave, and then it came, bleagh . . . the dog regurgitated what looked like a long red string, covered in puke, onto the grass. I knelt down and, with a gloved hand, picked up the offending item, which, it transpired, was a crimson-red suspender belt. As I held it aloft, the blood drained from the man's face. The lady looked at him and with absolute vitriolic condemnation said, *'That's not mine, George!'* She filed for divorce shortly thereafter – and took the dog with her. Both marriage and dog gone in one fell swoop.

This is an extreme, but there is little doubt that emotions are often laid bare in my consulting room. The cracks in relationships are often prised open in the emotional crisis of a critical illness or injury to a beloved animal companion. Often, one half of the couple loves the dog or cat, say, more than the other and this can expose issues in the relationship that are bubbling beneath the surface. I have been in a consultation where what started as a conversation about a dog has turned into a full-blown marital tiff right in front of me. I've even had a husband blaming me for his divorce, alleging that his wife fell in love with me – I highly doubt that and suspect I was an easy target for his anger.

When an animal who has become an integral member of the family is faced with a critical condition, it serves to highlight just how vulnerable we are underneath it all and can force us to confront some fundamental truths: what is and isn't important to our moral core; what we will and won't do when faced with a crisis; and how radically our reactions may differ to our partner's. Our ability to compromise and show compassion are often laid bare in such circumstances. These all lie at the bedrock of human emotional relationships but we rarely, if ever, have the temerity to air dirty laundry with each other unless forced to do so by a crisis – and that crisis sometimes happens in my consulting room. I think I am now pretty good at determining who will stay together and who won't!

Perhaps it has always been thus for veterinary surgeons because we have a glimpse into the inner workings of relationships through the conduit of our patient. Back in large animal practice in Ireland, I saw the dynamics of a very different marriage during another extraordinary regurgitation incident. I received a call from a farmer to attend a cow in difficulty with calving late one spring night. When I arrived at the farm, I found the cow collapsed with the womb side down in a very mucky yard. I lay down beside her in the shite, my waterproofs barely keeping the gunge from pouring in. After examining her, I realised there was no way on earth I was going to deliver the calf normally. The birth canal was too small and the cow was exhausted from labouring for hours. It was going to have to be a caesarean.

I trudged back to the boot of the car to get some kit, my wellies clinging to the icy muck and my breath hanging on the air. The light of the moon was eaten up by the sombre clouds above as the lady of the house drove the tractor up close so that the headlights would illuminate my 'operating theatre'. The sounds of cows and sheep in various states of restlessness filled the air with a cacophony of mooing and baaing as she got down from the tractor in her well-worn, long grubby skirt, which she shook at a noisy clucking chicken saying, 'Shush all of you now'. Miraculously the entire farmyard fell into a hushed silence. Her husband and I groaned as we tried to roll the cow over so that I could place my incision on her left flank. This side of the cow was covered in stinking, wet slurry and she was freezing cold and flat out. The miserable animal was in no condition to help herself, let alone to help us.

The farmer and his wife said absolutely nothing to each other, just nodded and gestured: a language without words. He grabbed a hose and sprayed the cow down, making her even colder, while his wife went into the house to fetch a couple of bedsheets and fill some buckets with boiling water. I joined her in the kitchen to sterilise my instruments in a saucepan of water on their range. The kitchen was strewn with the various accoutrements of cooking, living and farming. There was a tractor wheel leaning by the wall and items of clothing drying on a line tied between the window and a rail above the oven. Cups and pans and knives and forks lay in a pile beside a bath of potatoes on the table, and a dog huddled in an old coat at the fireside.

The woman didn't say much to me either, and when she did it was direct and to the point: 'There ya are now, plenty o' room for ya,' she exclaimed, as she moved a large soot-black kettle to one side on the hob and plonked a giant saucepan over the burning turf in the cooker below. I pulled back some old trousers on the line above my head and chucked my few surgical utensils into the water. 'Sure, if I'd a known ya had that little equipment I'd a got a smaller saucepan!' She gestured derisively towards the saucepan, as if the volume of my surgical tools might be an indicator of my surgical prowess. All of this was normal procedure when performing any operation on Irish farms at the time, but perhaps with a little less cynicism.

In fact, you don't need many instruments to do a cow caesarean, just a blade with a handle, scissors, some grabbing forceps to hold tissue, artery forceps in case of a big bleeder and something to hold the needle to stitch up at the end. I'd acquired a small dissection kit, wrapped in a green pouch, in vet school, to which I added, bit by bit, as the years went by. I had the same kit for my first decade in practice.

The farmer's wife and I went back outside and I crouched down beside the cow, shaved her flank behind the ribs as best I could with a blade, doused the area where I was going to make my incision with iodine, and rubbed it in, clearing whatever other debris I could in the process. Then I sprayed surgical alcohol all over the site, and the lady of the house, my newfound assistant, grabbed my steaming surgical instruments in their saucepan, and the sheets, which by now were also soaking in a bucket of boiling water. The farmer controlled the head end of the cow while I injected local anaesthetic along the nerves above my intended cut, though to be fair he didn't have much controlling to do as she was exhausted, the poor beast. Then he and his wife, working in perfect silent synchronicity, laid one sheet as a surgical drape and poured out my instruments from the saucepan onto the other, which was draped over the bale of straw that had been set as an instrument table.

The woman of the house and myself scrubbed our hands in a bucket of iodine water. In those days, there were no gloves, just bare hands – in fact, for my first few years as a veterinary surgeon for both large and small animals there were no gloves, just the power of iodine disinfectant and very short fingernails. The farmer's wife clearly worked hard on the farm; she had almost no nails on her fingers at all.

To stitch I used an instrument called a Gillies needle holder, an oft-maligned instrument that isn't used nowadays by many veterinary surgeons, who prefer to use a separate needle holder and surgical scissors to stitch and to cut the suture. The Gillies is a marvellous instrument with a needle holder bit at the tip and cutting scissors behind that so that one person can stitch and cut at the same time. As I was usually operating solo, with no assistant, it was perfect for me. I love my Gillies and I continue to use it to this day. She finally acknowledged the respect due to my meagre instruments by mumbling, 'That's a fine pair o' scissors anyway,' as she laid my kit out for me, and after a pause added, 'providin' that you can use 'em o' course!'

I cut into the skin just behind the ribcage, a so-called celiotomy or laparotomy. Then I put my hand inside. Damn! For whatever reason, including perhaps our rolling of the cow, the uterus was lying under the rumen, the largest of the cow's stomachs. I couldn't get the womb up into the incision and was battling against the rumen which was full of silage and gas. I had seen this before. In fact, I had heard of a vet who, unfortunately cut into the rumen instead of the uterus by accident.

I asked the farmer to quickly scrub his dung-covered hands and, with his wife's help, to try to pull the rumen back while I desperately tried to get the uterus into a position where I could make an incision. I tried and tried again, but I just couldn't get the womb up enough. The calf was too big, I wasn't strong enough, the giant rumen remained in the way despite the four hands pulling it back and at this stage we simply could not roll the cow over again. It was an absolute nightmare scenario.

Then, from the lane nearby, we heard the sound of singing – 'Di del didel didel do didel didel didel do', and on it went. It was the drunken, unmelodic voices of two local lads carrying loudly on the frosty air, as they walked home sozzled from the pub. The wife ran out to the lane and brought them in to help. They didn't care about the muck anyway, as they were well used to such a yard themselves. I got them to roll up their sleeves. They were nearby farming lads and had seen animals in such difficulties before; their neighbourly spirit rapidly kicked in and I now had four pairs of hands to help. I enlarged my cut into the side of the abdomen, while two pulled the rumen forward, one pulled on the skin backwards and one helped me to get the womb exteriorised.

Slowly, the womb started to creep up, just enough for me to make a cut in the uterine wall and grab a front foot through the amniotic sac. I cut into the sac and asked one of the lads to grab the foot. Any initial post-pub joviality evaporated with the sudden realisation that his contribution was central to the success of the operation. It was crucial not to pull the calf out too fast since I only wanted the minimum size of cut possible in the uterus wall, avoiding a straying jagged cut, which would make stitching it up a major pain in the arse, especially under the rumen. I asked him to 'hold fire' on pulling and to just keep the foot in place – which he did – as I reached into the bloody chasm for the other front leg. I held it fast while I got the head up enough to get a full pull on, simultaneously checking the size of the cut in the womb. When I was happy, I handed this leg to the second lad – who by now had also steadied himself a bit – and I grabbed the head.

'Pull. Pull now!'

And with that, as the lads lurched outwards and upwards to try to get the calf out, the second of them – without warning – rocked forward and heaved the entire contents of his gut around my sterile surgical site – Guinness, carrots, potatoes and whatever other unmentionable foulness was in there. I couldn't believe what I was seeing. As our friend slumped down in the muck, myself and the other lad were heaving in abhorrence and effort, while the farmer and his wife held firm, despite their hands being plastered with vomit and their faces creased with shock and disgust. We finally yanked the calf out.

'For fuck's sake!' his mate exclaimed to a chorus of groans from the rest of us. The calf was out and flailing around on some straw that the farmer had placed on the yard, mirroring the sick lad who was by now finding it hard to stand, much to the admonishment of his mate who exclaimed, 'What the fuck are you like, ya tosser?'

The farmer, his wife and I just stood there stunned, looking at the bloody wound in the side of the cow, now with vomit around it. I honestly had no idea what to say. The woman of the house grabbed a nearby hosepipe and started to wash the nastiness off the side of the cow, as I covered the wound as best I could with some large swabs. She turned to her husband and simply said, 'N' that's why I told you t'give up the drink. Bet you're glad now, aren't ya?'

I closed my nose and breathed through my mouth as she flushed and I tried to protect the wound. Her husband just looked at her and nodded silently. It was clear who wore the trousers, just as it was clear that this was their version of love. Finally, we got the cow cleaned up as best we could and all stitched up. The two lads lurched off home, the one continuing to berate the other. 'Ya fuckin' gobshite!' carrying on the air, as they drifted off down the lane. Despite everything, both the cow and the calf were fine. Another day at the office.

I have infections with even the most aseptic techniques nowadays, but those farmyard cows in Ireland often appeared to be immune to everything. I've stitched a cow with boiled-up strands from baler twine because I had no suture material and she was fine. I am also acutely embarrassed to admit, but when I was newly qualified, I once even inadvertently stitched my glasses inside a cow during a caesarean.

The cow was down, I was struggling and pouring with sweat and, because I was two-arms deep in the cow's belly, I got a farmhand to take my glasses off for me. He was struggling to hold the uterus out of the wound enough for me to stitch it up while the rumen and other guts were sucking it back in, so he must have chucked the glasses beside my surgery instruments near a big pile of gauze swabs. I must have flicked the glasses into the cow while I frenetically grabbed a handful of swabs to stop the bleeding and simultaneously stitched the wound and grappled with a big spool of suture material called 'catgut'. My attention was firmly on the womb because the incision I made had ripped, as the calf was being pulled out, and the torn edges were bleeding like crazy, so I didn't notice as the glasses must have fallen into the cavern of blood and got sucked under the guts and rumen. The farmer, the farmhand and I searched high and low and cleared out all the shed looking for the glasses but they were never found.

By then the cow was up and eating hay and I just thought that my glasses had been buried in straw and muck, so I managed to find a spare pair and forgot all about it. That was until about two years later, when one of the men who worked in a local abattoir told a cattle dealer friend of my dad that he'd found glasses in a cow, and of course the story got back to me! I am mortified to this day, but I simply did not know. God bless the sturdy bovine constitution.

Despite this, I was good at being a farm vet in Ireland, I think. I had great times, and a bit of lively banter with the farmers and their families. They were wonderful welcoming gracious people, for the most part, and cut from the same cloth as those I had grown up with, so I felt comfortable there. Still, it was time to leave and carve out a new path.

Back in Guildford, I was still operating without gloves, but with very well-scrubbed hands, one of the few things that my large animal and small animal practices had in common. I traded operating by the lights of a tractor for a lovely operating light in Mike Alder's practice. Of course, back in Ireland, things have dramatically moved on since then, and soon after I left, pristine new operating theatres for both large and small animals were built. David Smyth was not only a great vet, but also had great vision, and worked very hard towards his dreams, which, like my own, took time and money. I still had very little money and was saving for a new car because I'd driven mine into a river and couldn't get comprehensive insurance being under twenty-five years of age and too high a risk. So when I returned to the UK, I worked Monday to Friday at Alder's and took as many weekend jobs as a locum as I possibly could.

Sadly, as with the glasses inside the cow, I don't think I'd be honest with myself if I didn't confess one further inadvertent and innocent – but serious – mistake, in the hope that someone else in the future may avoid a similar debacle. I think it's probably best to just face up to the errors of the past, whatever the outcome and however well-meaning the original intent. I was locuming in a practice and a lady came in with her little girl and her Russian hamster, secure in a shoebox with holes punctured in the top. I asked what was wrong, trying to sound as professional as I could, given that I had never in my life seen an actual Russian hamster before. I was on my own on duty, so there was little I could do except my best in the circumstances.

'I think he's sick . . . he has a pink bit,' the lady replied.

I frantically searched the Filofax in my brain for the 'small furries' lectures at vet school, but had never heard of a 'pink bit'. I initially thought it must have something to do with his penis and she couldn't bring herself to say the word. I timidly asked where the pink bit was and she said that it was under his tail. Ah, that must be a rectal prolapse with 'wet tail', I figured, a common condition in rodents where they get a bacterial infection that can be caused by stress. The infection can cause diarrhoea, which may cause the hamster to strain to poo and then the rectum can pop out through the anus. Unfortunately for Mr Hamster, he was about to get a lot more stressed.

I reached inside the box to try to stroke him and have a look at what might be done. I asked the lady if he had ever bitten anyone, and she said, 'Good God, no, young man, my hamster has never bitten anyone in his life.' That was about to change: he bit me, hard. My instant response was to draw my hand back really fast – but, as I did so, he recoiled against the side of the shoebox and sadly, and quite instantly, the Russian hamster was no more.

The little girl just looked up at me with plaintive eyes. It was bar none, to that point, the single worst professional experience of my life. I didn't know what to say. Understandably, the little girl was crying and also understandably the lady was extremely angry. All I could do was apologise profusely and explain that Hammy had got stressed and then got diarrhoea, and then got more stressed and had a sudden heart attack when I inadvertently frightened him, and I was truly sorry – I had only been trying to help. I further quietly imparted to the lovely little girl that it was unfortunately really sad, but maybe for the best because he was so sick to begin with. It was truly awful and I'm ashamed to this day.

However, I firmly believe in facing the truth, and from my very first day in practice I made a decision to always give folks the facts no matter how challenging the circumstance – though I tried to be as gentle as I could with the poor little girl. Needless to say, I never went back to that practice again. I have since mended as many small furry animals as I could to try to make amends.

I had a few more consistently stressful jobs, but none as awful as that experience. Every time I became depressed looking at the long line of people queuing for the open surgery that was the norm at the practice at which I subsequently worked as a locum near Croydon, I'd say to myself, 'At least you haven't killed a hamster today.' Basically, if you turned up you would be seen, there was no appointment system, so I would consult all day from 8 a.m. on a Saturday morning until 8 p.m. on a Saturday and Sunday night – often not finishing until 10 p.m. – including being on call throughout the Saturday night. It was challenging. Then I'd turn up for work at the practice in Guildford on Monday morning, which by comparison was an organised paradise.

At another weekend locum job, also in London, the vet was so tight-fisted that he would only give me a choice of six drugs and five syringes with reusable needles to last the whole weekend. His precept was that all diseases of dogs, cats and rabbits could be treated with the contents of one of these bottles, or a few in combination. So it really didn't matter whether the problem was a tummy ache or a festering ear, the patient was going to get some combination of the six medicines I'd been given. I had a bottle of each, with a second back-up bottle if I ran out. There was penicillin-streptomycin, a broad-spectrum antibiotic, dexamethasone, an anti-inflammatory, Laurabolin, an anabolic steroid called nandrolone, Lasix, a diuretic called furosemide, as well as some multivitamin – which he gave to almost all patients – and of course Euthatal, which is pentobarbital sodium for putting animals to sleep. He was so tight that he got big bottles of cheap vinegar from a supermarket wholesaler and used it to 'sterilise' the syringes and injection needles to ensure multiple uses. The surgical kit, which was fairly basic, was stored in surgical spirit, as he hadn't bought an autoclave. The suture material was in one size only and con-sisted of a spool of catgut suture for internal stitches and a spool of nylon Supramid for skin stitches. One of the juniors washed the blood off the surgical swabs and hung them on a little line to dry so that they could be reused. Last but not least, even toilet tissue was economised: newspapers donat-ed for kennels were torn into strips and provided for 'our convenience'.

Another London locum job finished me off, though. I was working for quite an arrogant chap who figured he was a bit better than everyone else. One day I was about to pick up a scalpel blade to spay a bitch when I fumbled a bit, and in his own inimitable fashion he quipped, 'Wouldn't you be better off with a shovel, Paddy?' He was probably just joking and didn't mean to be offensive. And it wasn't the slur of being an Irish 'Paddy' that got to me as much as the fact that he didn't rate my surgical acumen at all. I was determined to do something about that.

I got out of locuming as quickly as I could, all my dreams still seemed very far away. On the upside, though, I'd met a lovely guy called Mark Havler, who was a countryside ranger, and I moved into the attic room of his house where I woke every morning to the sound of birdsong. At that house I met Andy Torrington, a surgical resident studying orthopaedics at the Queen Mother Hospital of the Royal Veterinary College. Andy explained to me what was involved in getting specialist training and I felt even more strongly that orthopaedics was for me. I'd always been inclined towards the discipline and I had seen first-hand what was possible when I was in America, but my chat with Andy crystallised that this was what I wanted to do with my life more than anything else. While I still didn't think I would be good enough, at least I knew what I would actually have to do to succeed, and I was then determined that I would give it my best shot. Andy was kind and helpful and I'm very grateful that he inspired me.

Having already been rejected for internships and residencies, I decided to get more veterinary qualifications and to study for the Royal College of Veterinary Surgeons Certificates in Veterinary Orthopaedics, and then Radiology. In 1992, I interviewed for, and got, a job with a veterinary group called Underwood and Croxson, which at the time had a large animal centre (today a vineyard) at Greyfriars, near Guildford, and several small animal practices dotted in various villages and towns nearby. I was a reasonable bet as a general vet, having had experience with all kinds of animals. I was also chatty with clients and think I garnered their trust. Having said that, both Mr Underwood and Mr Croxson were adored by their clients and could do no wrong.

I, on the other hand, could frequently do wrong. It was taking me time to find my feet as a small animal vet and I was frequently late for clinics, having rushed around the countryside between calls to sheep, cattle and horses. Back at the small animal branch practices, my nurses got the brunt of annoyed clients who were waiting too long for me and as a result they began to play some pranks on me. The primary culprits were Jenny, Jean and Becky. One day I rushed back in from calving a cow, ran down the corridor and grabbed my white tunic coat, pulling it on as I dashed out into the small waiting room and invited the next client in. I was perplexed to be greeted with astounded gasps and wide stares from all assembled. I followed their eyes downwards and found to my horror a condom with milk in the teat stapled to my breast pocket.

They played many other pranks on me, including taping clingfilm on the toilet, knowing I only had one pair of trousers to consult in which were then covered in pee. They jacked my car off the ground, took the wheels off, jacked it back down again on the wheels, now flat on the ground, and covered the windscreen with Shredded Wheat. (Apparently this was because I was always late and always hungry and would frequently delay clients to eat bowls of breakfast cereal.) Their fun with my cereal didn't end there: they hollowed out my Shredded Wheat and filled the biscuits with rabbit droppings – stopping me from eating them only after I had poured the milk and was about to tuck in. Oh, but their *coup de théâtre* must surely be the occasion on which they gave me two lovely jewellery boxes for my birthday. My little face was so excited gratefully accepting the carefully wrapped gifts, but my happiness instantly evaporated when I opened them to find a pair of rabbit testicle earrings and a necklace which, they gleefully told me, they had been hiding in the freezer for months. Those were the long-gone days before health and safety and other laws of decorum quashed such shenanigans.

On another occasion, the emergency on-call bleeper sounded at 6 a.m. There were no mobile phones in those days, and one had to call the bleeper service for the details of the call. 'Sheep hit by car on such and such a road between such place and such place. Immediate attendance please.' I jumped out of bed, leapt in the car, which at that time was always fully stocked with all I'd need for farm visits, and off I went, still wiping the sleep from my eyes. I arrived at the scene to find an inflatable sheep covered in tomato ketchup with one of my nurses perched up in a tree laughing and videoing the whole thing. So, as well as teaching me much medically, nurses throughout my career have continued to teach me the importance of a good sense of humour – albeit sometimes very much against my will!

We shared many amusing times, especially at the Christmas parties in a local hall, where we all got to see Mr Croxson dance to Right Said Fred's 'I'm Too Sexy' every year. Not that I can be too critical – my dancing hadn't improved from my days with the 'senior citizens' in Ballyfin Community Centre. The girls ridiculed my attempts to impress them with my John Travolta shapes, putting their fingers in their mouths to feign vomiting. I'd just tell them to shut up, and would carry on dancing the night away.

But unfortunately those same two words 'shut up' landed me in hot water and nearly scuppered my reputation before I'd even begun my further studies as a vet. An African Grey parrot with psittacosis, a lung and air sac infection, came into the practice for radiographs. We couldn't sedate or anaesthetise the bird for fear of killing him, so I had to hold the poor creature on the X-ray cassette, using lead-lined gloves and a lead gown – which radiation protection guidelines allowed at the time. He kept twisting his head and looking up at me and asking, *'What are you doing? What are you doing?'* I kept trying to keep him quiet, and maybe a few choice phrases escaped from my big Irish mouth in the process. We completed the radiographs, dispensed the medication and, as I was handing him back to the dear, sweet elderly lady who was his companion, he pinned his eyes, bobbed his head, stretched out his neck and promptly vomited on me. In African Greys, this is apparently a sign of love and affection because in the wild they feed their young this way and breeding pairs also do this as part of bonding. However, I very much doubt that's what he meant! Then he jumped up on the arm of the lady, craned his neck to one side and shouted as merrily as possible, 'Shut to fuck up! Shut to fuck up!' Thankfully, she was very hard of hearing and, even if she noticed, she chose to ignore it. The nurses, however, were far less accommodating and took great pleasure in reminding me at regular intervals. This was one occasion where I was grateful that a client was not listening to the animal!

Looking back now, like any other new graduate at the time, I was finding my feet for those first couple of years, occasionally slipping up, occasionally covered in vomit, but always meaning well and doing my best as I tried to carve out my future in veterinary medicine.

'Bless me, Father, for I have sinned. It's been thirty-five years since my last confession. I have used profane language, and I have inadvertently killed a hamster.'

CHAPTER TEN

Hedgehogs

The Prickly Truth

I love hedgehogs: I always have, and always will. I looked after my very first hedgehog when I was a child. I found one on the side of the road and kept it in the hay shed where I fed it until one day it was gone. I would like to believe that my hedgehog got well enough again to venture forth and go on its merry way. The very first animal I imagined that Vetman, my own personal superhero, fixed was a hedgehog that had both back legs chopped off, and he welded bionic springs on him with magic dust so he could jump stronger, faster, better, like the Six Million Dollar Man.

In Gaelic, a hedgehog is called a *gráinneóg*, meaning the 'ugly one'. Of course nothing could be further from the truth, not in my eyes anyway. To me they are the cutest animals on earth, so it was to my eternal consternation that I ran over one when I was driving to a lecture one night. I screeched to a halt and ran to its aid – I immediately identified that I'd broken the shin bone (tibia) of his back leg (for he was a boy).

A hedgehog doesn't generally survive in the wild with a broken leg because it can't scratch its ears to prevent ear mites, it can't run very fast from cars or predators, and even if it heals, it can have a leg that sticks out, meaning a fox can grab it, even when curled up in a ball. So I missed my lecture because I went straight back to the practice and fixed him instead. That was the first time I'd put an external skeletal fixator on a hedgehog leg, and I used a very narrow 0.9 mm pin to go up and down the bone lengthways to align the fracture, and very small pins through the skin from the outside, roughly perpendicular to the bone, two above and two below the fracture. Then all of the wires were bent over on the outside and enshrouded in a bolus of plumber's epoxy putty, which set rock-hard to hold everything together. It was kind of like a safety pin for the tibia. We nursed him for a few weeks, then removed the frame and sent him on his way through the undergrowth.

I've performed that operation many times since, once on four hedgehogs at the same time on *The Supervet*. I think that vets have a moral duty to give something back to the animal kingdom when possible without financial recompense. It's good for the soul. I'm acutely cognisant that facilities and staff wages come at a cost and, in the modern world, most things are monetised, but nevertheless, I think every vet was once a child with idealistic dreams of helping all animals, and even when life and other pressures take over, I think we should try hard not to lose that principle.

The only pressure on me at that time was working my way towards becoming a specialist. I studied whenever and wherever I could, at nights and weekends. When working for Underwood and Croxson, I had moved to live in a town near Guildford, called Ash Vale, and my favourite spot to study was under a big chestnut tree in Farnham Park. I saw several hedgehogs there and more than once, when I was feeling a bit stressed, I was visited by a robin redbreast, which, as always, brought me a smile.

Doing the work for the exams didn't bring many smiles, however, and I spent many hours at the Tongham branch of Underwood and Croxson sweating away in the tiny X-ray developing room, a cupboard filled with noxious chemical fumes from the vats of developer and fixer that we used for the manual developing of X-ray films. I was a perfectionist and was busy getting my casebook together for the exams, so I would survive all manner of torment to get the perfect radiograph. For both the orthopaedics and radiology certificates it was very useful to still be in general vet practice, since equine and bovine medicine was part of the curriculum. I spent many a night or morning sleeping in the service stations on the M4 en route to Bristol veterinary school or the M11 en route to Cambridge veterinary school, and also many an hour parked on the M25 trying to get to the Royal Veterinary College in London for lectures or courses.

I learned from anyone prepared to teach me. Stuart Carmichael and Simon Wheeler at the Queen Mother Hospital of the Royal Veterinary College helped me with my orthopaedics certificate and would feature prominently in my life thereafter. Mike Herrtage at Cambridge vet school and Francis Barr at Bristol vet school were both very kind and encouraging. I must have driven them crazy with my frenetic sketching of every radiograph and asking of endless questions in case I'd missed even the smallest detail. I sat beside Peter Van Dongen in radiology classes and drove him crazy too with my constant scribbling and nervous right-knee bobbing, but he became a great friend, evidently accepting my irritating habits as part and parcel of the idiosyncrasies that make me who I am.

I finally passed the examinations for both the Certificates

of Orthopaedics and Radiology in 1994 and 1996, respectively. Exams still made me sick with fear and worry even though I kept the most detailed notes, which I still refer to even today. The regulations were that I could take referrals having sat my certificate examinations, but I would not be considered a specialist until I'd taken further examinations, which didn't happen until very much later. Normally one would have one, two or three internships, sit certificate examinations and then do a three-year residency and write academic papers for publication to earn the right to sit for recognised specialist examinations. While working on several clinical projects for publication, I took concrete steps to try to conquer my fear of lecturing, which I guess may have been rooted in my childhood inadequacies. I enrolled in a drama school part-time and this certainly helped, but like my hedgehog friends, when faced with public speaking in a professional capacity, I wanted to just curl up into a ball and protect myself.

I was just about to give my very first public lecture in Rudgwick Village Hall, West Sussex, in 1997, when I felt a searing pain in my kidneys. I was bursting for a pee, and literally couldn't find the toilet quickly enough. I thought that I was just extraordinarily nervous. I was due to give a lecture on arthritis in dogs, having started to take some orthopaedic referrals after moving to Hunters Lodge veterinary practice in Ewhurst, Surrey, that same year. Philip Stimpson, who I had known from Underwood and Croxson, had bought it. This lecture was my first big foray into advertising my referral practice and delivering information of value to potential clients. I anticipated that around one hundred people might attend: clients of the practice, people associated with local dog clubs and friends I'd invited for moral support. Surely I shouldn't be this anxious?

Then, from outside the toilet, I heard two nurses from the practice giggling at me. I came out and berated them for rejoicing in my nervousness and went in to set up my projector. Each slide had been meticulously prepared but the projector seemed as jittery as me and kept slipping down the table, so I propped it up with the old tweed cap that I wore in general practice. 'Perfect,' I thought. 'Now if only I could stop peeing.'

The people gradually took their seats, and I hid behind the tatty curtains at the front of the creaky stage. I ran to the bathroom again – my kidneys were really aching I was peeing so much – and came back to commence the lecture. I got as far as the role of cytokines in the pathogenesis of osteoarthritis when I had to excuse myself again. I struggled through to near the end and, before any questions, had to visit the toilet one more time. I was exasperated, embarrassed and exhausted. It was only then that the nurses confessed that they had injected my banana with a horse dose of the diuretic furosemide. They could have bloody killed me. What were they thinking?! I don't think that nurses nowadays would attempt such a stunt, probably because they'd rightly be scared of being hauled in front of our governing body. But the only person who was scared that night was me.

Gradually I began to give more talks and lectures and my confidence grew, but it was dealt a major blow when I lectured to some vets and proposed a mechanism by which I thought elbow dysplasia might occur in dogs like Labradors. Historically, it was recognised that there was likely a poor fit of the three bones that made up the elbow, the humerus, radius and ulna, but the 'how' or 'why' wasn't understood. It was also recognised that there may be a primary developmental problem affecting cartilage called osteochondrosis.

The humerus is effectively supported on two pillars – the radius and the ulna – and the part of the ulna that meets the humerus on the inside of the elbow is called the coronoid process. The back part of the ulna, which we call the 'funny bone', forms a notch with the coronoid process into which the humerus sits like a saddle.

After having looked at the fragments I'd removed from diseased elbow joints during surgery, I proposed that the coronoid process cracked because of pressure overload in various patterns akin to an earthquake or an avalanche, like a butt cheek not properly fitting a saddle, and also the two parts of the saddle slightly moving relative to each other. I was pretty sure I was right, and proposed that the cartilage would wear away after the cracking, but not before – in other words, the pressure predisposed the cracks in the bone and that then cracked the cartilage. So I delivered the lecture and escaped to the bathroom (no diuretics administered this time – just nerves!). I was in the toilet cubicle when three vets entered and proceeded to berate my talk as the musings of a madman. Who did I think I was to talk about earthquakes, avalanches, butts and saddles at a veterinary scientific meeting? I just cowered in the toilet with my head in my hands.

It took me until 2006 to prove my theory by sponsoring a student at the University of Wisconsin to analyse the samples. When the histopathology slide came through on the computer screen in my office at 1 a.m., showing that the crack in the bone was indeed under a plate of initially intact cartilage, indicating that it wasn't a primary cartilage problem, I leapt for joy. I went on to publish many more papers on elbow dysplasia, and twenty years later I have helped to rename it as developmental elbow disease, which is probably a more accurate descriptor for this complex syndrome. To this day, it remains a pet subject of mine, and the information we've discovered has directly contributed to the innovation of many new techniques for treating this painful condition, some of which we have demonstrated on *The Supervet*. In fact, the average viewer of several episodes of the TV show probably knows more about this condition than I did when I qualified. In one paper that I endeavoured to have accepted for publication, a reviewer commented that I still wasn't allowed to use the geophysics of earthquakes and avalanches to describe the phenomenon in a veterinary journal, but in my view if we look hard enough almost everything is replicated in nature.

With clients I still regularly use the arse-in-the-saddle and the avalanche and earthquake analogies today, which they readily understand, but I also know that truths are constantly changing as new evidence emerges – so we only know what we think we know today. In medicine, much of what we know will change in a few decades, even a few years, so all we can do is be generous in imparting discoveries, thoughts and knowledge to the next generation, even if it turns out ultimately to be disproved, so that they can be better equipped to move things forward in the future.

I am indebted to all of the mentors, both in the UK and the USA, who have been generous and helped prepare me for the future. In 1993, I went back to America to attend the North American Veterinary Conference in Orlando, Florida, with my good friend Seamus from university. I was blown away by the sheer size and scale of the event. There were thousands of vets, and hundreds of lectures. I attended workshops on external skeletal fixation and fracture repair, and I was absolutely transfixed, even more than the plastic bones we had just transfixed with pins in the class. Afterwards, I tracked down some of the lecturers to beg or beguile them into letting me visit them to glean more knowledge from their capacious minds. I was insatiable. Seamus and I lay awake in the room of the Super 8 motel and dreamed how all of this knowledge would translate into the future, a future that for Seamus would involve building a series of very successful practices in Kent. It was also in Florida that I met Paul Manley, who allowed me to sponsor the project at the University of Wisconsin that led to the great elbow discovery. That's how knowledge works: share it and everyone wins.

I travelled far and wide in America over the following decade and tried to build my own training programme by learning from the person who I thought was the very best in their field. I had also met Dan Lewis at the Orlando conference and went to visit him at the veterinary school in Gainesville, Florida. There I learned how to put external skeletal fixators on real bones to repair fractures, which has helped hundreds of dogs, cats and hedgehogs since. I will never forget this world-renowned professor picking me up from the airport and driving me to a supermarket where he pushed my trolley as I got provisions for my stay. I was absolutely gobsmacked by his kindness and humility and Dan has remained a close friend to this day.

At Ohio State vet school in Columbus I learned from Jon Dyce, one of the most intelligent vets I have ever met, who also allowed me to stay at his home. Through Jon I met one of the godfathers of hip replacement in dogs, Marv Olmstead. The first time I saw Marv drill into a hip, pop some cement into the hole, pick up a plastic cup on his index finger and pop it into the hole, just eyeballing where it should be, and letting the cement set while chatting jovially to us, I was utterly fascinated. How did he know the correct angles and how to position it so exactly? Many years later, when I performed the same procedure, I genuflected to Marv in my head. At Ohio I also met Mike Kowaleski, who has become a lifelong friend and mentor, and I am proud godfather to his son, Nicholas. At Washington State University I met Russ Tucker, a godfather of MRI scanning, who has taken me under his wing in many debacles of diagnostic imaging, and at Rolling Stones concerts, too. There are too many people to mention who have encouraged me, mentored me, and shared their vast knowledge and friendship with me, so that I might become the best I can be. They all have a special place in my heart.

Every day remains a school day for me. I will never look in the mirror and think I've 'arrived' or I 'know enough', and I am acutely aware that I'm only as good as my next surgery. I think most of the great surgeons are not arrogant, and many of the arrogant surgeons aren't so great. I have tried to repay the kindness shown to me by sponsoring fellowships, internships and residencies at the universities where I have been inspired, and I'm more proud, by a million miles, of their achievements than I am of my own. The student at Wisconsin who studied the elbows with me has gone on to become a specialist, as has a student who I sponsored at Florida and three more at Ohio State, with another nearly graduated as I write. Seeing them lecture with confidence, intelligence and truth fills my heart with pride.

A huge moment for me was when I gave my first lecture in America at the Veterinary Orthopedic Society meeting. I was probably more nervous than I had been in Rudgwick Village Hall – but I wasn't peeing as much, thank God. It was the first time I had ever used a laptop, since every previous talk I'd given had been with a slide carousel. I had no idea how to present properly, and I suppose I must have rushed through 120 slides in twenty minutes. Everyone in the audience was bewildered. Then a lady stepped up to the microphone in the middle of the hall to ask a question. I suddenly realised it was Gretchen Flo, a much-revered professor of orthopaedics and co-author of Brinker, Piermattei and Flo's *Handbook of Small Animal Orthopedics and Fracture Repair*, a bible for budding orthopods. I was about to be buried in my own ignorance, and I wanted to curl up in a ball and disappear. Gretchen just leaned into the microphone and said: 'Doctor Fitzpatrick, we were all sitting here down at the back and we have no idea who you are, or where you've come from – in fact we have no idea what you have just been talking about – with it being that fast 'n'all . . . But we were all just wondering – what kinda coffee do you drink?'

God bless America and God bless Gretchen! By not asking me a difficult question, she had by default given the go-ahead for my acceptance into the community. Another fellow nearby muttered, 'I've no idea who he is either, but I'd follow him into battle any day.' It was by no means a stellar performance, but a huge weight had been lifted off my shoulders. In a subsequent year, I won the prize for best presentation at this meeting. I rang Mammy all excited to tell her, but such things registered little in the overall scheme of life. She said to me that was 'nice', to take care that it didn't go to my head and, more importantly, to wear a hat so as not to catch a cold 'out in all of that snow' in Colorado. She added that she had, that week, seen a kingfisher bird land on the windowsill, something she had never seen before – and wasn't that a wonder! Every wonderment is relative, I have learned, and my mammy never fails to remind me to keep my feet on the ground – and my head in a hat, rather than in the clouds.

In October 2018, almost exactly twenty years since that first lecture, I shall deliver a keynote speech at the American College of Veterinary Surgeons symposium. This is the biggest honour of my professional career, and I really hope that Gretchen will somehow vicariously delight in the irony. I'll try a slightly slower delivery and hopefully not feel so much like a petrified hedgehog. I'll also reduce the amount of water I drink, and maybe wear a hat on the day before – just in case!

I moved to Hunters Lodge primary care veterinary practice in 1997 and set up a referral service taking animals from other surrounding primary care practices that needed neuro-orthopaedic surgery. The practice owners, Phil Stimpson and his wife Delia, were very kind and supportive. I continued to take inspiration and encouragement from wherever I could and Willows referral specialists in Birmingham and Davies in Bedford were particularly influential. Andy Miller and Malcolm McKee, two men who were working as hard as I was, sat me down one day on the stairs in Willows and told me exactly what would be needed if I wanted to make it in the referrals world and if ultimately I wanted to become a specialist. Richard Whitelock and Jerry Davies were instrumental in me passing my radiology examinations. The prospect of becoming a specialist was daunting but I decided to plough on.

The Hunters Lodge practice was in the middle of the countryside, in Ewhurst near Rudgwick, and to begin with I was involved in farm animal work as well as primary care small animal practice. What the practice lacked in size, we made up for in the magnitude of our dedication and compassion, but it was a small place with a tiny waiting room, two consulting rooms and an office that was built as an annexe onto a dwelling house. The 'surgery', which also doubled as the preparation room and X-ray room, was a garden shed out the back of the annexe, the X-ray developer was in a small wooden hut where I also took phone calls if they were private, and another wooden hut served as the kennels, where there weren't very many spaces, so we needed to get patients in and out relatively quickly. We didn't have room to swing a cat, which I little need to emphasise is neither ethically nor legally acceptable!

I still had only a beeper pager to rely on, which sounded randomly day and night. On one occasion, it bleeped at about 6 a.m. to call me out to lamb a sheep at a nearby smallholding. In the sunny early morning breeze, I walked up to knock at the imposing door of a beautiful country house. A lady of about forty years old, whom I'd met at the practice before, opened the door and directed me to where the sheep was in a nearby outbuilding. She then asked me to pop by the house afterwards as there was something else she wanted me to take a look at. The lambing was easy, just a head down in front of the pelvis and I got it out in no time – job done – and innocently headed back to the house as instructed.

I knocked on the door, which opened to reveal the lady in her dressing gown, with some rather racy suspenders and a rather fancy basque beneath. She just smiled and asked if I wanted a cup of tea. It appeared that she and her husband were not getting on too well and she had hoped I would fill the void, as it were. I declined the cup of tea on the basis of strict professional ethics, of course!

Gradually, as I became increasingly bonded to the small animal practice at Hunters Lodge and took more and more referral work from surrounding practices, I had fewer farm calls to attend. One of my final call-outs was to an articulated truck carrying about three dozen cattle that had overturned on a flyover bridge at the junction of the A31 and the A3. One beast was hurled onto the motorway below and other cattle were badly injured, panicked and mutilated and they had to be shot. Fire crews cut the roof off the truck to release the rest of the cattle. It was disturbing, an absolute massacre that sealed the fate of my large animal days.

An era was drawing to an end for me and I was becoming increasingly frustrated that neither farm animal practice nor general small animal practice lent itself to advanced surgical intervention. Usually the only options were to fix the animal relatively simply, or put the poor creature to sleep, so I continued my training and my efforts towards becoming an orthopaedic specialist. My early efforts were less than impressive, as was my early toolkit. I performed my first few dozen spinal surgeries with a Dremel wood drill covered in a sterile wrapping, and my orthopaedic bone drill was a Makita from a hardware store, also covered with a sterile wrap. On one occasion I was holding a tibia bone with my left hand and, while drilling through one side with my right hand, I hadn't realised the other side had cracked with the fracture. I kept the same pressure on the drill, but there was no other side to the bone and so it went straight through my left hand.

'*Fuck!*' I could see the drill bit poking out of the back of my hand and blood filling my glove. Instantly, I made the decision to reverse the drill and pull back while the shock still numbed the pain. It was fairly acute – but fortunately the drill bit had bounced between two of my metacarpal bones and I was OK. I wrapped the hand tightly with Vet Wrap, a multipurpose cohesive bandage, and finished the op, since there was no support surgeon for back-up. Thankfully it was a clean spike-through and the injury healed fairly quickly.

Inspired by all of my educational trips abroad and by the world around me, I developed thought processes, and mainly did good work with those trusty tools. For example, I developed an external skeletal fixation system for the pelvis of cats based on the principle of a grappling hook, whereby the grabbing pins suspended the fractures from above and held everything in position, while the fractures healed without any plates or screws. The first ever cat I used this technique on was called Cheddar, and I vividly remember that it was a sixteen-part fracture, and that plates and screws just wouldn't do the job because the pieces were so small and the hip socket was shattered. So I developed dissection windows and realigned everything with the pins like chopsticks down a well, before securing them in place. The cat looked like my beloved hedgehog in the end, but the operation was a success.

One day I operated on a Doberman that was affected by 'wobblers disease' or caudal cervical spondylomyelopathy syndrome, a sad and debilitating condition with many varients, which I've had an avid interest in for my entire career. Basically, for this poor dog, a couple of discs in his lower neck were bulging due to degeneration, causing compression on the nerves to the front legs and the spinal cord as well, making the back legs wobble because the signals didn't get through properly. The dog was paralysed in all four legs and had to be carried everywhere. At that time, we had very few surgical devices with which to intervene, and the clients had limited finances, and therefore had no option for referral elsewhere. In fact, even if referred, there remained a paucity of device options. I carried out a procedure with one of the few disc spacers that were available at the time, a solid metal washer, which I inserted between the vertebrae in place of the discs. The Doberman, however, did not regain the use of his legs and, with huge sadness, I had to put him to sleep.

On the drive home from the practice later that day, I was quite tearful and pulled the car over into a lay-by to regain my composure. It was December and it had begun to snow a little, well more like sleet actually. Through the hazy white, I looked across the road towards a yard where a man was loading Christmas trees into a horsebox. The horsebox was enclosed with four rigid sides so when it was full, it was full; there was no piling another one on top. The man stared quizzically at his loaded box; he had one last Christmas tree in his hands. Then he stuck the pointy end of the Christmas tree into the tree trunks already loaded, and pushed and pushed until it wedged in there by prising the others apart and compressing their branches a bit more, no doubt. *Eureka!* A Christmas-tree-shaped intervertebral spacer was born. I spent the next decade or more perfecting a spinal fusion system, which has now come to fruition and is called FUSS – the Fitz Universal Spinal System. It uses various sizes of titanium Christmas-tree-shaped spacer devices to drive between vertebrae, pushing them apart when the discs have collapsed or the vertebrae have become deformed. Much later, I got the idea of joining sequential Christmas tree spacers together for disease in adjacent disc sites using an upside-down saddle plate screwed to each spacer – based on the saddle of a horse – and linking each of the saddles with dumbbells – inspired by my visits to the gym – so that I could fuse multiple sites in the neck of any dog affected by this disease.

I came up with lots of other ideas in that hut at Hunters Lodge practice but did not have the technical wherewithal to realise their application until many years later. I think that

I learned this art of innovation from my father. Daddy was the king of improvisation and I was delighted that he did once visit this little practice in Ewhurst where he had a first glimpse of what I might do as a specialist vet, and I felt proud showing him how I performed a fusion of the wrist in an injured dog – with my wood drill to take the cartilage off the joints and my builder's drill to make holes for the screws of the plate. I told him about the drill bit through the hand and he reminded me of picking turnips with him, musing that he had trained me well for pricks in my hands. I also told him about the criticism of my lectures. He smiled and again reminded me that when enough thorns go in, you feel the pricks less. Maybe he was the king of hedgehogs too – prickly on the outside but soft on the inside.

During this part of my life I got to choose my own new family too. Stuart is my physiotherapist whose weekly ministrations have been as important psychologically as they have been physically for me over the past twenty-five years. I have suffered numerous injuries in the course of my life and work, but it's the wear and tear that takes the greatest toll. Ironically, orthopaedic and neurosurgeons wreck their own bodies through bad posture, constant hunching for hours on end and unusual movements, causing within themselves the very problems they are trying to fix in a patient. Stuart generally comforts, offers some sagacious advice or just tells me to 'get a grip!' I was with Stuart on 13 February 1996 – when I heard Gary, Mark, Howard and Jason on the radio telling us that Take That were splitting up. I was a big fan – but as was his vocation, Stuart was a voice of reason in the darkness!

I met my close friend Rick, a better-looking version of Rod Stewart, when training at the gym in 1992. We've shared many laughs together through the years, including the time

I jumped out of a cardboard birthday cake dressed as a surprise 'lady' for his fortieth. I looked like a hedgehog because I had ripped my stockings, wig and dress with my false nails; Edward Scissorhands had nothing on me! I also went in search of hedgehogs with Rick on the last proper holiday I took, which was in 2000, to Australia. More specifically we set off in search of echidnas, which look like hedgehogs, and platypuses, which look like nothing on earth. We had black plastic bin liners on our heads with torn-out little eyeholes so we could see as we huddled in the rain of the jungle near Cairns. Three hours passed as we hunched silently in the undergrowth until we finally saw both creatures. I now love hedgehogs, echidnas and platypuses. Though echidnas resemble hedgehogs, actually they are egg-laying mammals and, together with the platypus, are the only surviving members of the monotreme order.

The sad reality is that humans threaten all wildlife, including our humble hedgehog. Hedgehogs have changed little over the last 15 million years, yet they could be totally extinct within fifty years. While I've been alive, 95 per cent of all hedgehogs in the UK have disappeared because of pesticides, decimation of hedgerows and road traffic.

My childhood hero Vetman, whose first patient was a hedghog, wanted us to realise that we need to look after all of the animals in the world. I have had successes and failures, I have made mistakes, I have looked in the mirror and I have sought my own truth in large animal practice, small animal practice and now specialist practice. The more I understand about the prickly truth of where I have come from and where I want to go, the more I realise that I might spend my entire life publishing papers, giving lectures, passing exams, innovating, receiving criticism and praise, looking after animals who are loved by families, and even potentially feeling 'important' – whatever that means – but I may die without translating the one undeniable truth that is so hard for anyone to really take on board in the middle of our busy lives: animals do *not* get a fair deal in return for all that they give to us, and we are destroying their homes. We do so at our peril. Within two or three generations, we may have a planet ecosystem that has collapsed.

My dream is to translate the love that we feel for animals in our homes to love in their homes too – wherever that may be and whatever form that takes. I knew even back then in the 1990s that I wanted to translate 'listening to animals' who are part of our families to a wider responsibility for all living creatures. I had overcome my fear of lecturing, but for this, I would most certainly need to take on a far bigger challenge: to learn how to communicate on a much wider scale – and that's when the *drama* really began.

CHAPTER ELEVEN

The Swan and My 'Son'

Life Imitating Art

'How dare you have an actor pretending to be a vet on a wildlife programme and killing a swan,' read one of the letters of complaint from an angry television viewer.

On 2 April 2005, I had in fact been a vet pretending to be an actor on BBC 1, in the TV hospital drama *Casualty*. The following night I was a vet, actually being a vet, and pretending nothing at all on Channel 5, in a programme called *Wildlife SOS*, where sadly I had to put a swan to sleep. On the BBC drama I had said 'safe journey' to my 'son' as he was dying, and on Channel 5, back in real life on the wildlife programme, I said something similar as the swan slipped away, and a few dozen innocent viewers thought I was an actor masquerading as a vet. One can't really blame the viewers for a little confusion: art and life really were imitating each other.

Perhaps I got the role on *Casualty* because I was the only actor in the audition who could actually pronounce 'subacute sclerosing panencephalitis'. In the episode, I was helping my son to die by overdosing with drugs, and Imogen Stubbs, who played my on-screen wife was, unlike me, a very talented actress and brilliant at crying at exactly the right moment. I wasn't. However, I did invent the word *'povickimise'* which means to cry false tears – since I had to rub Vicks ointment in my eyes to do so.

When I settled in Guildford in Surrey, I'd not only moved with the dream of expanding my veterinary knowledge, helping more animals and ultimately specialising. I'd also harboured a secret dream. It wasn't the kind of thing one vocalised in Ireland in the eighties: I wanted to go to drama school. I couldn't get that affinity with literature and poetry I'd felt since secondary school out of my head, nor did I want to. I yearned for the chance to explore what great writing, films and theatre meant in the real world and why they transported me to another level of awareness, insight and perception. I wanted to understand how the emotional connection between page and performance actually worked and why it really mattered in the world, in *my world*.

To this day, I think it's unlikely that I would have come up with inventions or solutions to surgical problems if I thought purely in scientific terms. I have felt more alive when listening to music, or watching a play or a film, and I have found scientists more interesting when they painted pictures and did not just draw in straight lines. I think that most scientists who have great insights have an artistic bent. I think that, even back then, I also knew instinctively that if I wanted to make a difference to animals on a global level then I was going to need to understand how words worked, and especially spoken language in the media.

Towards the end of 1993, I was spaying a small dog at the Underwood and Croxson practice in Tongham, Hampshire. I planned to send the dog home that same day, but the lady couldn't pick her up because she was going to the theatre. On the phone, I asked her in passing if she was going to see something nice, and she said that it was a play in a small theatre in nearby Farnborough at which she often helped out. She said that her dog liked it down there too because she got fed. I was intrigued so I found the address and one day decided to cycle down to check it out for myself.

I parked my bike outside 75 Guildford Road East, and checked if I had the right place because it looked like a normal residential house. Yes, indeed, this was it. I walked towards the front door but a sofa and some carpets blocked it, so I went to a side door and just as I was about to knock, I spied another entrance down the alley in the garden beyond. I didn't knock. I was mesmerised by the apparition of red Chinese trellis shrouded by deep purple curtains, and some kind of Chinese dragon emblem on the doorway leading to what looked like a hybrid of a Victorian theatre and a Chinese circus, with lanterns hanging within. Entranced, I quietly went in and inside found a dimly lit, musky-smelling, velvet-seated, curtain-shrouded cocoon. This was Farnborough's Prince Regent Theatre.

From an alcove to the left of the stage, a tall slender man with a bald head and a kind smiling face emerged from the half-light. He bowed under a low lintel and walked towards where I was standing, in the central aisle, between the old-world velvet and dark-wood chairs. 'Can I help you?' he asked. This was Philip Gilbert. Neither of us knew it then, but he would help me more than anyone before or since.

Philip and I had an easy rapport from that very first handshake. This little theatre had been his partner Freddie Eldrett's lifetime dream. Freddie had been a dancer in a number of West End shows and had persuaded Philip that they should build a small seventy-seater theatre to allow young aspiring actors the opportunity to work with professional actors, receive an education and maybe get a break into 'the big time'. The Prince Regent Theatre was an ornate shed that glowed like a Tardis in the garden of the house they shared together.

Philip Gilbert was born in Canada and appeared in many theatre productions, including some in London's West End before being hired by J. Arthur Rank to star in the 1961 British western *The Singer Not the Song*, starring Dirk Bogarde and John Mills. Under contract to the Rank Organisation, he appeared in many films during the fifties and sixties, starring opposite Peter Finch, Norman Wisdom, Stanley Baker, Bob Monkhouse and Donald Sutherland, to name a few. His stories were the stuff of legend, such as hanging out with Marlon Brando and James Dean. He knew what the *real deal* was, and what wasn't. He was the real deal, but he was the man who you never really saw – generally, the character actor who turned up, did his thing and left. He was also an invisible talent in the seventies, when he played the voice of the computer TIM in seventy or so episodes of Thames Television's cult hit *The Tomorrow People*, and again in the radio plays in the early noughties. He was happy being second fiddle, never hogged the limelight, and was a rock of sense and support for so many people, particularly those who needed it most. He was selfless and one of the kindest human beings I have ever met.

When he came back from America, he and Freddie set up home in Great Missenden in Buckinghamshire. It was reputedly an idyllic existence in a beautiful cottage and they lived near Roald Dahl, who Philip chatted to from time to time. Apparently Roald told a great anecdote about Winston

Churchill who, one day, was walking in a field nearby. Maybe he was visiting Clement Attlee who had a home there. The story goes that Churchill passed a bull tied to a post in the ground by a chain through the ring in his nose. Churchill allegedly quipped, 'He may live a life of inordinate boredom, but at least it is punctuated by moments of ecstasy.' Philip enjoyed recalling this gem, though I doubt he ever saw the parallel with his own life, since he had given up this wonderful retirement existence to help Freddie to achieve his dream. Early on I realised that he was shackled to that theatre for better and sometimes for worse.

It was a dream that ultimately destroyed Philip, but ultimately saved me. After stumbling across his theatre, I had signed up for a drama course and immersed myself in its teachings. As Philip drowned in the financial and managerial burdens of owning and running a struggling small theatre, he saved *me* from drowning in myself. I had a head full of dreams but none of them seemed to have any hope of being realised. I recognised that I wasn't skilled enough as a vet and wanted to specialise, but I was having no luck getting any internship or residency; I knew that I wanted to build a great vet practice, but, at this time, it was still just a pipe dream; I wanted to try to change how the world respected animals, but I didn't know how; and I realised that I yearned to understand theatre and drama, yet I didn't fully know why. I felt like I was right back at the start again and that I would not amount to much.

Philip was my primary tutor and in between rehearsals for Eugene O'Neill's *Long Day's Journey into Night*, we'd chat. One evening, we were sitting on a bench, on the small patch of grass between the theatre and the house, under a blossoming apple tree, and I explained my predicament as best I could. In the play, James Tyrone bemoans the waste of his life when he believes he could have been a great actor, and I said something along the lines of: 'So, the thing is – I wanted to be a vet since I was a child, but I'm so frustrated that I can't move quicker and make a bigger difference. I find some kind of comfort or peace in literature and music, and I love to escape inside the theatre here. I'm confused and I don't know the reason why.'

Philip just smiled and said: 'Noel, it's fine to be confused, it's fine not to know the path exactly, it's fine not to know the reason why – but what you really have to do is find a reason big enough.'

These wise words changed my life forever. From that moment on I was searching for *my reason big enough* and it fuelled everything that happened on the road to building the practice, my field of dreams – where *The Supervet* is today filmed.

Often during lessons, Philip would hold an imaginary camera while teaching me how to communicate more effectively. It wasn't about acting, he said, it was really about communicating – delivering the words with integrity and sincerity. Some of his most important lessons taught me how to use the stage or the TV screen to communicate truth, to lift the words from the page and make them matter, at least for a moment in time, and hopefully long in the memory thereafter. If I hadn't met Philip, and if he hadn't believed in me, encouraged me and taught me many vital skills for life, I am convinced that *The Supervet,* this book, or possibly even Fitzpatrick Referrals itself, may never have happened.

I had an old record player and I listened over and over to John Gielgud, Richard Burton and Laurence Olivier ply their trade. I was absolutely fascinated by how, with mellifluous voices alone, they could transport the listener to another time and space and world of emotion. I studied and rehearsed with great enthusiasm for exams with the London Academy of Music and Dramatic Art (LAMDA) and with Philip's expert tuition, on 24 July 1995, I was awarded a gold medal with honours. I had never enjoyed exams before, but this was a whole new experience – and I loved it.

I'd been studying at the same time for certificates in veterinary orthopaedics and radiology, and for those few years I spent more time asleep in my car somewhere, after or before going to lectures and theatre rehearsals, than in bed. I'd work during the day as a vet and most weekends too, except when I was performing, and either finish early or take the weekend off for the matinee and evening performances. I knew exactly what I was aiming for – an understanding of art and science – but I readily admit that learning stagecraft, character creation and analysis of literature came much easier than learning scientific facts. Theatre was food for the soul and I had an insatiable appetite. I also realised that it gave me a much better work–life balance.

With Philip, I went on to discover Ibsen, Chekhov, Shakespeare and many other great writers. We performed in pantomime together at the Prince Regent Theatre; he was Mother Goose and I was the Demon Discontent. He had a wicked sense of humour that bubbled to the surface more than occasionally. There was a scene in which the Demon Discontent was looking in the magical mirror while Mother Goose held it, and every night he wrote something more and more rude on the glass. Luckily we were playing for laughs.

One matinee performance saw two busloads arrive – one carrying some ladies from a retirement home and the other bringing children from a local primary school. Throughout the first act there was a very vocal child in the front row and his sole objective seemed to be upsetting the actors and reducing the enjoyment of everyone else around him, so that he himself would be noticed. He did this by randomly shouting obscenities, rudely heckling everyone who came on stage, throwing sweet wrappers around and putting his feet up on the low proscenium at the front of the stage. Needless to say, many of the old ladies were horrified whilst most everyone else was distracted, but not necessarily by the magnificence of our performance.

It was therefore my distinct pleasure to scare the life out of this child as we came on for the second act. While coercing my reluctant little helpers to steal Mother Goose's golden egg, I asked, 'And do you know what I want you to do?' At this point, I was to put my hands on their shoulders, one to either side of me, and volley forward towards the audience with my next line. This time, though, I jumped down from the stage into the auditorium, straight in front of the naughty boy, and added, 'I want you to get your smelly feet off my stage!' His horror wasn't the best bit – that was afterwards when an old lady came up to me and thanked me for the great excitement.

On another occasion, the thanks were a little more poignant and showed why I yearned to understand what it's like to translate words into emotions and feelings. In *The Supervet* now, the integrity of real-life dilemmas, love, hope and despair are translated. The truth is that if I just talked about medical techniques in scientific language throughout the programme very few people would watch it. It was never intended to be a programme about science; it was intended to be about hope and love. I often get accusations from both within and outside of my profession saying, 'It's put on, it's pretend', but I can categorically tell you that there's nothing pretend about it – it's real life, love, pain, loss, fear, happiness and, critically, peace and redemption.

If I lost my integrity for one second, I have lost my soul, and if I lost my soul or the reason I do any of this at all, including this book, then all is lost. If all of this was for my ego alone, then I would be morally bankrupt and it would all be worthless. Part of the reason that I now treat the camera as a friend on my shoulder is because Philip taught me that truth is everything, and it was in his theatre – and not the operating theatre – that I realised by travelling these journeys together, with honesty, we could and would make the journey better for all of us.

One night, Philip and I were in a workshop performance of Ibsen's play *Ghosts*. It is a harrowing play about a boy called Oswald, who is suffering from syphilis inherited from his licentious father, whom he had worshipped, and, to make matters worse, he falls in love with his half-sister and is rejected. Philip played Pastor Manders, the priest character, and I played Oswald who is dying from his disease and from heartache. The climax of the play centres on Oswald's mother, who must decide whether to help her son to die with an overdose of morphine. This was a profoundly difficult play for me because as a vet I use morphine all the time, and I knew tragic cases of vets who had in fact taken their own lives. I had not, as yet, suffered the heartache of lost love then, but that would come in time.

After one particular performance in front of a small audience, a lady came up to the stage door. She was sobbing while she thanked me. I asked why she was crying, and she revealed that her son had died of AIDS. She said that the performance had, for the first time, helped her to come to terms with her grief, helplessness, pain and loneliness. Through this brief encounter I came to understand the power of truthful communication. That was what I had been looking to understand – and I finally did.

The last play that Philip and I performed together was called *Gaslight* by Patrick Hamilton. Philip played a detective and I played a young man who was driving his wife mad by making her think that she was imagining the gaslight in their house was dimming when, all the while, he was in the attic using the gaslight to look for the jewels of the old lady who'd previously lived there, and whom he had murdered. Unbeknown to me, during this time Freddie had become increasingly jealous of my friendship with Philip. He was drinking a lot and, although there had been a few snide remarks, I didn't realise the full extent of his dislike for me until one night in rehearsal just before the show opened. Freddie was the sound and lighting technician for the play. At one point in the first act the gaslight is supposed to dim as the detective walks on; however, suddenly a bright spotlight was shone right in my eyes and Freddie roared tempestuously, '*You fucking c***, you stole my man! You fucking c***!*' Philip was understandably distressed and I was speechless as Freddie stormed off. Later that night, Philip's bedclothes and mattress were chucked out on the path beside the house.

We finished the short run of that show and not long thereafter Freddie forbade me from coming to the theatre or ever contacting Philip again. Philip was unbelievably kind and considerate, and understandably didn't want to hurt Freddie or me, and so he acquiesced. The degree to which Freddie felt threatened by my friendship with Philip was intense, as was the enduring love they shared, so with a very heavy heart I knew that it was my responsibility to resolve the situation by walking away. I could not conscience either Philip or

Freddie being hurt. I feel quite sure that the termination of our friendship must have been as hard for Philip as it was for me. To this day I carry the empty void of the loss of his life-transforming companionship. For many months I felt a huge mix of negative emotions, but with time came understanding and acceptance, and now all I feel is tremendous gratitude to Philip for enriching my life. Hardly a day goes by when I don't think of my confidante, mentor, inspiration and dearest friend.

Philip and I had a favourite rehearsal spot under a giant chestnut tree near Guildford and I treasured those moments. There wasn't the slightest bit of the self-consciousness that had permeated my entire existence to that point. The work we explored set me free and allowed me to be whoever I wanted to be, especially myself. One of Oscar Wilde's poems, 'To My Wife', was a favourite of ours:

> ... If of these fallen petals
> One to you seems fair,
> Love will waft it
> Till it settles on your hair.
> And when wind and winter harden
> All the loveless land,
> It will whisper of a garden,
> You will understand.

Philip understood absolutely. He was patient and calm, always with his kind smile, his hand on my shoulder when I desperately needed someone to believe in me – just as I was, not as they expected me to be. He encouraged me beyond measure and his final act of faith in me was to write to many casting directors on my behalf asking them to meet with me for various productions. I found one of his letters and was really humbled and more than a bit tearful about what he wrote:

I have worked with Noel for five years and he is one of the most unique, versatile and truthful actors I have seen. His outstanding background, academic qualifications, personality and appearance, coupled with vocal and physical power, earns him the opportunity in my view to excel in our profession.

One such letter was sent to the casting directors of *Bally-kissangel*, a programme made for the BBC in the UK and RTÉ in Ireland. The character I was hoping to audition for was called Danny Byrne. An actor called Colin Farrell got the part and played it well from 1998 to 1999. I think he's done all right for himself since!

Another letter went to a casting director called Malcolm Drury in 1998.

'Allow me to be frank at the commencement – you are not going to like me.' These were the very first words I said to Malcolm during my first audition for him in Hammersmith, west London, in October 1998. It is a line from a play called *The Libertine* by Stephen Jeffreys, a play I was, eighteen years later, due to attend with him in the West End, but he died suddenly, aged seventy-two, and was buried a few days before our planned night out.

Despite my opening line, Malcolm and I not only liked each other, we were great friends for all of that time. He was an old-school casting director and a magnificent champion of young actors. He made journeys to theatres in far-flung places across the country every week to see small productions in order to spot new talent, and he kept a Rolodex of actors in his head so he knew exactly who to contact when a part came up that matched their talents. He would never cast just from a headshot and a videotaped audition. Much later in life, he never coped with the computer age and steadfastly refused to use a mobile phone – he didn't agree at all with the modernisation of acting, and the pitch of a single video online rather than meeting the actor in person. He once told me that Catherine Zeta-Jones turned up to audition for him when he was casting *The Darling Buds of May*, and he told her to go away, clean up her punk look and come back with a nice dress and a nicer attitude; she did – and the rest is history.

Malcolm cast everything from Laurence Olivier's *King Lear* in 1983, to Rik Mayall's *New Statesman* in 1987, and was head of casting at Yorkshire Television until 1993. Then he regularly cast *The Bill* and *Heartbeat* and introduced me to many directors for whom I auditioned. I starred in both shows twice: as a vet searching for a poisoner of crows and as a sheep rustler in *Heartbeat* in 2000 and 2002; and in *The Bill* as a shady dog dealer and an even shadier drug dealer in 1999 and 2001.

The first time I auditioned for *The Bill*, Malcolm leaned over and whispered, 'That wasn't quite right now was it – can you try to feel it just a bit! Shall we start over again?' At the audition for the vet in *Heartbeat*, the casting director on the project called him and said that I didn't look like a vet. Malcolm had great pleasure in saying, 'He is a vet, you fucking idiot.' Interestingly, years later, when I came to pitch *The Supervet,* the producer at the time said the same thing to my friend Jim, with whom I filmed the pilot. I wonder what a vet actually looks like in people's heads. Ironically in

Heartbeat, I was actually acting being a vet and there were no complaints!

Heartbeat was my favourite show to work on – we were out filming in the very beautiful countryside of Goathland in Yorkshire. I sat in the caravan studying my veterinary notes, and had a lovely time chatting to the actors on set. I learned lots of things, including a very good lesson on humility, which I take with me to this day. One of the actors was Bill Maynard who played the very popular comedy character Greengrass on the programme. He firmly believed he was the star of the show, which I suppose to a large extent he was, and one time I gave him a card for his birthday with a picture of us standing by a sheep inside it to remind him in case he'd forgotten who I was and he gave it back to me with an autograph! He was always lovely to me, and I'm sure he meant nothing but kindness – but the episode did remind me to keep my ego in check. Over the course of my time as an actor, I came across some who were genuinely humble about the hand fate had dealt them, and others not even that adept at pretending to be.

Humility was something Caroline Dawson, who eventually became my agent, also instilled in me. I'd been introduced to her through Malcolm and she did not tolerate big egos, so that suited me well as I never felt remotely good enough to have cultivated one. If someone was being an arse, she'd tell them outright. She didn't have time for complainers either, which, coming from my daddy's farm, also suited me just fine. She also liked dogs and she liked me, so we got on very well indeed. She was, in her day, a formidable force of nature and stood up for me more than once. She wasn't shy about telling people what she liked, so one did well to stay firmly inside the realms of her benevolence.

Malcolm also didn't pull any punches about actors' indulgences. We'd often sit in a theatre watching a play and he'd nudge me and say something like, 'He can't even read the fucking line, let alone act it', or equally insightfully, 'He was all right wasn't he – but would probably be better if he could relax a bit and take the pole out of his arse.' We bantered and laughed like an old curmudgeonly couple. He did not suffer fools – he just told them to get over themselves. He hated facades almost as much as he hated the red tape that got in the way of getting the job done – he saw it and he told it as it was. I got upset easily, taking the rejection at auditions deeply personally, while other actors seemed to be able to shrug it off. I guess that's because I never felt good enough at anything.

Both of us were therefore particularly pleased when I got my first chance at what felt like a proper film role as Crawford in *The Devil's Tattoo* (which was also released as *Ghost Rig*; 2003). It was big in Japan, apparently! We were all young actors trying to do our best, even if it isn't the greatest film or the best acting from me – but still, it was a main character in an actual film and I had an absolute blast. This experience also taught me three important lessons about life. Firstly, nothing is ever work if you're laughing. I had the best 'holiday' shooting this film in Scotland. Secondly, life is all about the choices you make and the work you put in; several of the cast went on to be very successful in their careers, and I made some big decisions too, which, in the end, worked out OK. Thirdly, be grateful for what you have because it can all be gone in the blink of an eye. In the film, I shot a gun and when the bullet hit the target a squib exploded, which was like a tiny stick of dynamite with a small explosive device in it. A tiny shard of plastic shot out, bypassed a protective

Perspex screen and hit me just to the side of my left eye, which swelled up like a balloon. If it had hit a few millimetres further over, my career as a surgeon could have ended even before it had rightly begun.

Malcolm and I were laughing about this as we walked along the South Bank in London, a spot that Philip and I had also loved, because we often went to the theatre there, and Malcolm reminded me that 'it can all be over in the blink of an eye'. We were sat on a bench looking out on the Thames in silence, just listening to the hazy vibrations of the city, taking in the view before going to see a show at the National Theatre nearby. I had been talking about big worries I had at the practice, and he just listened. He pulled the cigarette out of his mouth, where it was more often than not, and still looking out at the river, and as if talking to the air, he continued, 'The things you worry about are all passing, you know. You only hold onto them in your head. Don't get attached to the physical things, they don't matter. It's what you think of "yourself" that matters – cos that might stop you doing bigger things.' Then he paused, took another puff of his cigarette, and added, 'Chase your dream – as long as you're doing the right thing – even when nobody is watching.'

Malcolm was always honest with me, but incredibly kind with it. I remember keeping him on the phone spilling out more woes of some kind. He gave nothing but stern admonishment and a reminder that it was all in my head. Later that night, I came home to find a small bunch of snowdrops in tinfoil on my doorstep. He had come all the way from London by train and back again just to make me smile. I love snowdrops because they pop their heads out of the coldness to tell us everything's going to be OK, that there's hope. He often sent me cards with snowdrops or cherry blossoms on, and in later years, when I got too busy to keep in touch with the world of drama, he religiously sent me newspaper cuttings every week of all the things he felt that I might have liked to see had I not been so busy.

The last acting role I did before I hung up my thespian cloak in 2007 – literally in this case as my character did wear a cloak – was a movie called *Framed*. I played a detective, Inspector Beckett, investigating the theft of a Rembrandt painting. The film was set in Mansfield and Oriel colleges in Oxford, which were beautiful locations, and I had a magnificent time. It was a low-budget film and the acting was questionable again on my part, but apparently the film, which came out the following year, was popular in Hungary. What with *Ghost Rig* being big in Japan, I guess you could call me an international film star!

The best thing about *Framed* was that I got to act opposite Robert Hardy who played the provost of the university in our film, but much more importantly played the vet Siegfried Farnon in the BBC TV series *All Creatures Great and Small* (1978–90). He kept forgetting his lines, so I became of use to him and we got on well for the few days we were there. I was totally enthralled while in his company, and wanted to hear every story he could remember about being an actor playing a vet, in the days before health and safety rightly stopped the actors from sticking their arms up cows' wombs in order to pretend to deliver calves, or pretending to have a crack at stitching up or dehorning. Robert was full of wonderful stories, and I hung on his every word.

I had grown up watching *All Creatures Great and Small* and, like many vets I know, the programme directly influenced my perception of what it might be like to be a vet. In the late 1970s and 1980s, throughout Ireland and the British Isles, young people viewed veterinary medicine through the eyes of a particular Yorkshire vet, James Herriot, and in no small way the programme helped set my ambitions for *The Supervet* many years later. When I set out to make *The Supervet*, I wondered what it might be like to give children who might wish to be vets a looking glass into the future for the profession in the twenty-first century. Judging by some of the letters I receive from children nowadays, thankfully I may have positively influenced some young minds. For me, it's a truly wonderful feeling, to see inspiration growing in young people who yearn to take the message of love and responsibility for animals onwards into the future, just like James Herriot inspired me.

In *All Creatures Great and Small*, Siegfried Farnon was based on real-life vet Donald Vaughan Sinclair, who was apparently even more eccentric than Hardy portrayed him. Sinclair took his own life with an overdose of barbiturate on 28 June 1995. Sadly, the suicide rate in the profession is still high by comparison with other professions, and of course it happens for many reasons, though some, no doubt, are related to stress and easy access to drugs. *The Supervet* tries to show accurately and honestly some of the challenges, difficulties and stresses associated with the veterinary profession. Veterinary practitioners, like workers in any other profession, can benefit hugely from occasions where they can come together in a community of understanding, support and compassion. I strongly believe that, as a profession, we should look after each other better, as we do in our vocation of looking after animals. Because I am acutely aware of the positive impact such a meeting of minds can make to an individual, I created an event called the VET Festival (VetFest).

VetFest is an education and wellness event for all veterinary professionals, including vets, nurses, physiotherapists and other associated disciplines, where we bring together experts in different aspects of veterinary medicine from all over the world to lecture and share their knowledge and experience. We host them in tents in a field with yoga, mindfulness and mutual support as the integral core. A party atmosphere augments the learning experience, good food is served and there are people wandering around dressed up in silly costumes, and playing guitars sitting on bales of straw dotted throughout the field, and at the end we have a fabulous party with great singers and bands. Every veterinary professional likes to hang out with his or her peers, we like the respect and the camaraderie; we like to feel we're making a contribution; we like to feel part of something special. While I appreciate the value of conferences in hotels and other venues, I wanted to take a more holistic approach that merged what we love to do with what we need to do: education and entertainment. I have had some of the best times of my life at Reading or Glastonbury festivals, so my thought was: why not make education fun, too?

My hope is that VetFest will become an annual Glastonbury for vets, vet nurses and vet professionals of all kinds, where we help each other to cope with the stresses and strains of veterinary life and openly share ideas, successes and failures for the greater good – a tangible community of compassion. I think sometimes as veterinary medical professionals, we feel that we must have a particular kind of 'persona', but as a result we can lose touch with the fact that we're just people trying to do our best in sometimes difficult situations. VetFest is a way of acknowledging that we are all in this profession together, and so we should be as kind and considerate as we can to each other, with an ethos of mutual respect, no matter what level we're at.

VetFest is a tribute to all of the people who inspired, supported and encouraged me – people like James Herriot, but none more so than Philip and Malcolm. They allowed me to understand that there need not be a dividing line between art and life, one need not imitate the other – they can co-exist and both can be real, when truth and integrity are at the core. Sell out on either for one second and all can be lost.

There came a point where I needed to make a firm decision: to either take the acting more seriously or quit because auditions were getting in the way of me being the best vet I could be. I really enjoyed my time as an actor, and if I had the time I'd do it again in a heartbeat, every pun intended. I might have got better had I stuck at it, but I couldn't be master of everything and I had learned what I needed.

The world of acting was very tempting, especially when I got down to the last two or three people for interesting roles in movies or TV that would take me away for several months at a time, but the potential for the Avengers of my childhood comic books to join Vetman and assemble to save the animal world had long been my overarching dream. Everything that I had done to that point had been to prepare me for their great adventures that lay ahead. I realised the time had come to focus on pursuing my ambitions and dreams as a vet. I knew it would take me fifteen years at least to become a proper specialist and build the kind of practice that was needed. I was prepared to do whatever it took in terms of hours committed and discomfort endured. I was no stranger to hard work and I knew that what I was about to do would consume my life completely.

I set out to find a home for a referral veterinary practice, to be available twenty-four hours every day of the year and ultimately to use what I had learned with Philip and Malcolm to build a platform to try to make a real difference in the world. Both of them had believed in me even when I didn't believe in myself. They wanted the best for me and didn't judge me; they allowed me to be whoever I wanted to be and were content to walk the journey without expecting anything in return.

It wasn't until many years after we'd very sadly lost touch that a friend told me that Freddie died in November 2003 and Philip slipped into a coma and died on 6 January 2004, aged seventy-four. I miss him so much – his selflessness, integrity, compassion, courage and faith. In 2007, just before I moved to the practice in Eashing where *The Supervet* is filmed, I planted a chestnut tree for Philip. I had grown it in a pot from a sapling taken from the tree under which we had rehearsed many years before, and I had carried it with me through my two previous practices. Now, finally, the tree had a resting place at Eashing, and I planted it outside my office window so that I could remember Philip and my 'reason big enough' on a daily basis.

Years later, I was attending the TV Choice awards in September 2016 at The Dorchester in London. I'd just got out of the back of a taxi, in which I had changed out of my surgery scrubs because I'd come straight out of an operation, and sauntered in. *The Supervet* was up against Paul O'Grady's *For the Love of Dogs*; stiff competition, so I had gone to show the production team some support, anticipating the outcome. On my way in, I bumped into a successful actor who Malcolm had discovered and had given his first job to because he could ride a motorbike. I rang Malcolm the following day to say thanks for giving people a chance, but there was no answer. Later that day, a friend called to say that Malcolm had died suddenly – in the blink of an eye, as he had himself predicted. I was absolutely distraught. That evening, I picked up a voicemail he'd left me, saying he couldn't understand a single thing I was doing on *The Supervet*, but it was wonderful and he was proud and happy for me.

I planted a cherry blossom for Malcolm beside Philip's chestnut tree on the day after he was buried in October. Very strangely, on that same day, it was drizzling with rain, and as the sun came out there was a rainbow. Then something else extraordinary happened: a small robin came and landed nearby. I ran inside, welling up with tears, to get my phone to take a picture. By the time I returned, the robin had flown off – with Vetman I like to think – but miraculously a second rainbow had appeared, and at the ends of each were the trees I had planted for my dearest friends who had nurtured my dreams. I captured this picture for all of eternity – my own personal treasures at the end of the rainbows.

I had two paving slabs laid outside the National Theatre overlooking the river, each with Malcolm and Philip's names, so that, side by side, they can walk there with me forever.

'Don't allow what you think of yourself to stop you chasing your dream' ...

'All you need is a reason big enough' ...

Life doesn't need to imitate art, nor art imitate life. Life is art.

Thank you Philip and Malcolm for teaching me these precious lessons.

CHAPTER TWELVE

Birdbrain Takes Flight

The Hut in the Woods

Every Saturday morning from 2000 to 2002, while I was working at Hunters Lodge veterinary practice in Ewhurst, I was up with the larks – no small feat for a night owl like me. On these Saturdays, though, I wasn't up early to get back into the consulting room. I have never felt that being a vet should preclude someone from pursuing any other profession or dream they want, be it a rap artist, an actor or a radio presenter. I refused to be pigeonholed then, as now, and so when the opportunity arose to present the early morning Saturday breakfast show from 6 to 9 a.m. on BBC Southern Counties Radio, I jumped at it. I can't rap, by the way!

I was really enjoying my foray into theatre, television and film, but radio has an intimacy, spontaneity, truth and a real conversational context that you just don't get from the written word, prerecorded television or film or rehearsed theatre. As a radio presenter, you get to speak to people you'd never normally come across in everyday life, and tackle some big real-life subjects or just banter about trivia. It involves a whole different skill set which I was very keen to learn. Just like with my drive to study drama, I really wanted to understand how to operate a mixing desk, how to collate thoughts to present a coherent radio show and, most of all, I wanted to further learn how to communicate: how to talk to and get messages across to a wide audience on a big platform and how to make a show that would be thought-provoking and entertaining at the same time.

As with my academic and drama pursuits, I sought out a mentor, and I was fortunate to find one of the best in the business. Neil Pringle still hosts the weekday breakfast show on BBC Sussex Radio and is a hugely gifted radio broadcaster of immense integrity who knows what makes good radio, a craft that needs to be learned through actually doing the job and experiencing the highs and lows. I feel extraordinarily fortunate to have been allowed to do just that on his watch. He was considerate, funny, patient and generous with his time and his talent.

I loved everything about working in radio. After a late night in the practice on the Friday, I was often totally knackered and would turn up exhausted on the Saturday at 5.15 a.m. with a bundle of weekend papers I'd picked up from the newsagent's on the way, but within ten minutes, and a couple of instant coffees, I'd be devouring the newspapers and buzzing with adrenaline for the show ahead. I went on-air at 6 a.m. on the dot and, for the next three hours, I got to play my favourite music, which was all on CD in those days. Working the analogue desk is an art form. The digital desk came in just as I was going out the door, but I'd love to give that a whirl someday, too.

The Saturday morning breakfast show covered current affairs, interesting stuff in the local news or papers and politics. I was completely impartial on all subjects – colour, creed, race, religion and sexuality, infamous or famous, I treated all the same and still do – which played to my advantage. I tried to listen to people with an open mind, without judgement and with more than a bit of compassion. This was to prove particularly important when it came to outside broadcasts covering highly competitive local events such as dog shows, weaving and knitting competitions, topiary or, most particularly, the lawn bowls local league competition.

I was once on an outside broadcast covering a bowls tournament. As a bystander, the matches look so calm and serene, but when they heat up, I don't think I've ever witnessed such competitiveness, heightened emotions, combative spirit and raised tempers. I was actually slightly scared! Craft fairs proved to be equally hazardous, especially if a small coterie of ladies in my fan club were waiting to meet me. On one occassion, I innocently found myself embroiled in a heated debate about the winner; I was lucky to get out alive. I learned lots about dealing with live 'incidents' on Southern Counties Radio, and a fair amount of on-the-job crisis management. I was on-air on 9 February 2002 when the sad news of the death of Princess Margaret came down the wire. All normal programming went out the window and interviews and related commentary came in. It was an interesting time of intense learning in broadcasting which would later stand me in good stead for live television.

The prize for the regular competition phone-ins in the 'Early Bird Club' on my show was Noel's Hug Mug, a much-sought-after and highly desirable item for any household. The mugs were made by a local pottery in Grayshott and I have to say they were pretty special: an artist drew my hands and this image was then printed onto the mug so that my fingers were wrapped around it and my thumbs were behind near the handle, as though hugging the mug. Inside the rim was my catchphrase: 'Waking you up on a Saturday morning'. Only a hundred of Noel's Hug Mugs were ever made and I still proudly have numbers 01/100 and 13/100 (for my birthday!). I often turned up at the house of a winner to have a cup of tea with them, sometimes recording our chat with my trusty fluffy microphone and tape box.

On one such occasion, I arrived to find a lady still in her dressing gown. She let me in, all delighted, and I thought she was just a bit overexcited for the Hug Mug delivery, but in fact she had been feeding a pigeon with a broken wing in a shoebox and asked me if I would take it back to the practice and fix it. She was such a lovely lady, I felt honour-bound, and so I did. I brought it back to base, taped some lollipop sticks to the sides of the broken wing and looked after the pigeon until it was ready to be released a few weeks later. This dear lady had brought literal meaning to the 'Early Bird Club' and Vetman would have been proud of me.

The referral work was ramping up in Fitzpatrick Referrals, which was still a part of Phil Stimpson's Hunters Lodge practice, so I had to give up the radio show because of even later nights at work. In early 2003, I relocated to the new branch on Woodbridge Hill in Guildford. Although clients had to park in the carpark of the nearby pub, the Wooden Bridge, the new premises were a major step up from the huts in Ewhurst, even if the space was still small and the preparation room had to serve as the scrubbing room, the autoclave room, the X-ray room and the minor procedures room. We still had a very limited number of kennels and I often consulted early in the morning and operated until well after midnight, seeing dogs out late to make space for the next patients.

I brought one of the Hug Mugs to the new building with me, and kept it in a small cupboard under the stairs where the X-ray developing machine was housed. This machine was an improvement on dunking the films and developing by hand, but was still quite a noxious dark place to be locked in while loading and unloading the X-ray films from cassettes, and I needed the coffee to keep me sane – and awake. The operating theatre had been newly built and was lovely, plus there were two nice consulting rooms, although the location next to the kebab shop was unfortunate. I grew sick and tired of hearing people make the same joke all of the time: because we were next to a kebab shop, it was 'in one door, out the other' for my patients, which I found very offensive. Admittedly, it wasn't the ideal spot for a referral practice but Phil was always very supportive and I'm grateful that he allowed the embryo of Fitzpatrick Referrals to grow there.

I look back on those days and nights next door to the kebab shop in Guildford between 2003 and 2005 with a mixture of fondness and frustration. Ironically, it was only a short walk from the practice where I had started out with Mike Alder when I had first come over to the UK ten years earlier. Once I had determined my 'reason big enough', I was more desperate than ever to build my own practice, but it still seemed very far off. I did have the good fortune to have one of my early mentors, neurologist Simon Wheeler, come work with me, and we had some good times together. However, I got turned down for planning permission at locations a couple of times and I didn't have enough money anyway, so all I could do was continue to invest my time and energies in scientific contribution and working with like-minded individuals in pursuit of future academic advancement in orthopaedics and neurosurgery: one can't aspire to build the best veterinary practice in the world if it has no core based in factual science. That would be like building a Ferrari without an engine.

I was still travelling to the United States to both attend and deliver lectures at veterinary conferences. I was feeling more relaxed about lecturing and beginning to enjoy the buzz of scientific endeavour and the acknowledgement of colleagues. I would take on every lecture slot I was offered at a conference, without any clue as to how I was going to get the notes and the slides actually done in time, generally having worked seven days a week at the practice in the run-up. I have given well over a hundred lectures in America over the past fifteen years or so and I have never, ever gone there with one completed. I have written lectures on my laptop in planes, trains, automobiles, toilet cubicles, nooks and crannies in conference centres and any nest I could sit or crawl into, but most of my lecture writing has been done in hotel rooms across America. I have never given a lecture without preparation, but I have come a cropper once or twice and delivered below par, which I feel bad about for letting folks down, but generally, just because of the sheer numbers of cases I have presented – the implications, successes and failures – I have brought useful material to the table.

I can say without ego and with confidence that during the ten years between 2003 and 2013, I likely operated more cases in ortho/neuro surgery than anyone else in the world. I was often operating seven days a week and it would have been physically impossible to operate on more patients than I did at that time unless one actually didn't need to sleep. I frequently worked through the night sorting out patients and also frantically pulling together, in a folder on my laptop, all of the radiographs, CT scans, MRI scans and operative photos I needed to construct some kind of narrative for my lectures. I was without a doubt pigeon-eyed with exhaustion, sometimes having not slept for thirty-six to forty hours before getting on a flight. I would crawl onto the plane, get to my seat and be 'out for the count' in minutes.

I generally arrived at my destination in the early evening and started lecturing the following morning, so I had a finite number of hours to plunder the images in the folders on my laptop and bring the lectures to life. I have been to many cities and seen none of them, just the inside of a hotel room, which all look the same, and the one thing the vast majority of American hotel rooms have in common is tubs of Pringles potato chips in the minibar. For more than fifteen years, this Pringles routine has been part of my coping mechanism: upon arrival at my hotel, I hurl my bag on the floor; pull the chair back from the table; take out my laptop, plug it in and boot up; take off my trousers, as I always write best in my pants, and head straight for the minibar. I open a pack of Pringles and lay out the potato chips individually, or very occasionally in pairs, all over the room – on the bed, on the bedside table, on the window ledges and even in the bathroom, to encourage me to get up and stretch to get the treat. Every half-hour of lecture writing by the 'Pringle clock', I allow myself to get up and eat a Pringle. This helps to focus my lecture writing and also sets a countdown clock in my brain.

From experience I know that there are between twenty-four and twenty-six chips in every 50g can. This is of course significant if one is writing lectures to the time of the Pringle clock as the treats need to be rationed and distributed according to the length of time needed to write on any given night. So, if I need to write for ten hours, that means one crisp every half-hour and a bonus four, or maybe even six, at the end. Sometimes, as I go up to the room in the elevator,

I longingly hope for two tubs of minibar Pringles as then I can go with the more indulgent option of two crisps every half-hour, which yields twelve hours of writing, with or without a bonus two to four at the end. Occasionally, with only one tub to hand, I have taken the risky option of setting the clock to get all lectures done in six hours – which means two crisps every half-hour. *Whoopee* – a veritable feast! Of course, once the lectures have been written and delivered, great fun is to be had on end-of-conference nights across the globe – thankfully with superior nutritional content than available in hotel minibars.

For whatever reason, I think that my lectures have been better accepted in America, Europe, Australia and Russia than in the UK. The same is true, I think, of the veterinary reception to the procedures shown on *The Supervet*. A few years ago, I was again in a toilet cubicle after a conference in the UK and it was déjà vu from fifteen years earlier. I had just delivered a lecture on customised implants and I started by saying that I believe that the veterinary profession has a moral responsibility to explain each of the various options for every implant surgery we offer, regardless of whether it is mass-produced or custom-made. I said that any implant system can have complications and we can all fail. The guys having a pee at the urinals were criticising my approach, saying I was pontificating and being patronising. Similarly, just a year ago at a conference in America, I was in a queue for coffee and overheard a delegate from the UK being highly critical of a lecture I had just delivered on a new technique to surgically treat lower back pain in dogs. At the same time, a US delegate came up to me and thanked me very much for my contributions.

It's not all plain sailing when one genuinely, for all the

right reasons, wants to move veterinary surgery forward, but everyone has a right to their opinion. Nevertheless, I remain open to explaining why progress is essential but must be carried out in an ethically robust and supportive framework. Change will happen anyway: as a profession we have a collective moral responsibility to progress, just as our human medical colleagues do. In fact, our human medical colleagues generally use experimental animal models, including dogs, to ensure efficacy, safety and evidence for drugs and implants. As this is indeed happening anyway, I feel that the veterinary profession needs to ask why we would not want to look at a framework where we collaboratively move veterinary medicine forward with an attitude of mutual respect for the greater good of each other and the animals we serve. We are all accountable for what we say and for what we do.

Attitudes in the veterinary profession are changing, though, because society demands the best level of care for our animal friends and expects our profession to give people all of the options, even if they do not choose those options. It is also critical to maintain our reputation in society as professionals whom the public can trust to do the right thing. However, I don't think there's any place for overindulging in our own self-worth and thinking we're great just because we have passed exams, or we are professors, or we have an impressive practice, or we've delivered great lectures or scientific papers. At the end of the day, we are all fallible, we all fail and, when we do, we have to accept that we're only human and just doing our best. We should be as kind as we possibly can to each other.

I was certainly fallible when I had to go to Moscow in 2013 to deliver several lectures. I was seriously considering not going at all, having come down with the flu from hell. I rang the organiser to explain and a heavily accented voice echoed back down the line, 'You come to us, or we come to you!' The choice was clear: if I didn't voluntarily get on the flight as planned, they would come and get me on a plane. I got on the flight and, as soon as I was through customs, I was greeted and whisked off in a van where I was immediately plied with various kinds of potions to ingest, along with lotions to sniff and rub on my chest and throat. Before we got to the lecture venue, I was taken to a room, laid on a bed and given acupuncture and massage, then more lotions and potions. The effect was transformative: I was ready to begin. I lectured for eight hours straight, with two half-hour breaks, to a conference hall so packed that there wasn't even standing room at the walls. I kept trying to close the laptop and say I was done, but the organisers repeatedly opened it up again and asked me to carry on. There were two people simultaneously translating alternating statements from me as I rattled through. They could not get enough knowledge; we finished close to midnight, though they still asked for more. At the end, they gave me a children's poem that is apparently Russian folklore for a kind of Doctor Dolittle, and they hailed me as such. This was their highest honour and I was deeply touched.

Back then, in 2004, I was certainly no dignitary when I sat with my bank manager in the Wooden Bridge pub on Woodbridge Hill in Guildford, and drew my view of the future on a napkin. The bank manager was less than helpful: he said I was a birdbrain, that I was away with the fairies, looking for too much money and that the risk was too high. I explained my vision for three hospitals: one for orthopaedics and neurosurgery; one for cancer and soft-tissue surgery; and one for advanced stem cell regenerative bionics, because I felt that in the future we'd be able to rebuild body parts. I may as well have been asking him to take me to Mars.

It was futile to argue: the bank wanted to lend me some money because that's how banks make a profit, just not enough money – because that's how dreamers make dreams happen, not how banks deal with risk. I was despondent because I couldn't find a way to build bigger premises to house Fitzpatrick Referrals. Then Falcon came to my aid.

Martin Patrick brought Falcon, a black Labrador, into my surgery on 29 December 2003. He was nearly paralysed following an acute intervertebral disc extrusion. The spine vertebrae are like train carriages between which the discs act as buffers. Each buffer disc is like a jam doughnut, and when they dry out they become less spongy and can either bulge their dough (annulus fibrosis) outward or leak their pulpy centre (nucleus pulposus) through the dough. (Both are called 'slipped discs' by some, but because the disc does not 'slip', it's not a term I favour; nor can either form of disease be 'popped back in'.) In Falcon's case he had the latter, which can yield an explosive clump of jam coming out and hitting the spinal cord at a rate of knots, often causing rapid or progressive paralysis. We needed to operate fast.

Falcon's dad, Martin, an avid Arsenal supporter, left Falcon in my care while he travelled to an away match in Southampton. Arsenal and Falcon both won that night, Arsenal 1–0 retaining the FA Cup, and Falcon his mobility. That season Arsenal went on to win the Premier League, were hailed as 'The Invincibles', and notched up 49 unbeaten league games, but sadly Falcon had a complication with scar tissue and I had to operate a second time. Thankfully Falcon recovered and went on to enjoy the beautiful game of running around a field. Perhaps I wasn't such a birdbrain after all! Unfortunately, beautiful Falcon succumbed to aggressive cancer about a year later, but I shall forever be grateful to him and to Martin for coming into my life.

During our journey with Falcon together, observing my dispirited mood, Martin wondered if it was due to the failure of the first operation. I confided that this wasn't the cause, as I was in fact optimistic for Falcon's chances after the second operation, but not for my chances to obtain new premises. A few days later, in early January 2004, Martin introduced me to a farmer called Peter Stovold and they took me to see a derelict farm on Halfway Lane in Eashing, Surrey. I remembered that several years previously when I had been working as a general vet, I had attended a sheep with a prolapsed womb in one of the sheds on this site. Thankfully, I was talented with regard to all things sheep-related, and there were no bad memories for the farmer.

There were four old buildings on the plot of land constructed from a variety of brick and cement, asbestos, metal girders and corrugated-iron roof sheets, which in the case of one of the buildings, a hay barn, had blown down and was imploding. Some of the trusses holding this barn up were so rusty that they, too, were near collapsing point. Old plastic drums, rusting bits of farm machinery, ropes, chains, broken pallets and all manner of debris was strewn across the site. I love the movie Field of Dreams and from the moment I set foot on that land I knew that was what I had found: my own field of dreams. Once I had seen those buildings I was determined that this farm would be the ultimate home for my surgery. I dreamed I would perform the most advanced surgeries to save animal lives that the world had ever seen, where twenty years earlier I had saved a sheep. I think my daddy might have approved of that transition after all

– bringing the animals and the hope back to a derelict farm. There were just a few small obstacles – money, planning permission, endless stress and very many sleepless nights.

I knew that it would take years to get planning permission to make the build in Eashing happen, even if it were possible, and it might not be. I had only a small amount of the money needed, which I'd managed to save from operating at Hunters Lodge. I couldn't begin to afford to start construction without a massive bank loan. So I needed to find a job where, if I worked hard enough, I could generate enough revenue to encourage the bank to lend me more.

The bank I had been with since a student in vet school and all through the nineties had refused to back my proposal. I went to another bank manager and asked him how much he would give me as a loan based on what I'd already saved. I found premises that I could convert relatively cheaply into a temporary vet practice in Tilford, a village outside Guildford. During the following ten years, I went through four banks as each, in turn, declined to lend me what was necessary to make the ultimate dream happen. I remain in substantial debt to this day, but back then all I knew was that I was ready to work day and night, seven days a week, for as long as it took to get there.

The three men instrumental in allowing me to build the next stage were quantity surveyor Peter Morgan, lawyer Jack Marriott and estate owner Lance Trevellyan. When I borrowed the first tranche of money, Jack commented, 'they have the shirt off your back'; at the second tranche, 'they have you by the balls'; at the third tranche, 'they have the trousers off your arse'; and at the fourth, 'they have your pants and you are butt-naked, Noel'. I'm very grateful for Jack standing by me all these years.

When Fitzpatrick Referrals moved to Greenhills Estate in the beautiful village of Tilford in Surrey on 11 December 2005, two days before my thirty-eighth birthday, many people called me far worse things than a birdbrain and a fool, saying it would never work. Clients would need to drive into the middle of a wood, down windy country roads, onto a rural estate eight miles from the A3. The naysayers said nobody would ever come. I had the voice of doubt on one shoulder telling me I was a fool and the voice of optimism on the other saying, *'Go right ahead – you have a reason big enough and you're doing the right thing.'*

It was an absolutely necessary, but always intended to be temporary, move. The site in Tilford was a Canadian army barracks during the war. Surrounded by trees in the middle of the woods, it was a wooden building, within which we constructed two operating theatres, two consulting rooms, a few offices, a prep area, an X-ray room, two operating theatres, some kennels and a nice reception area. We began with fourteen people including nurses and receptionists. I just needed somewhere that I could accommodate more surgeries and more kennels for a few years while I was trying to obtain planning permission and get enough money together to build my field of dreams at Eashing.

On many days, I saw a herd of deer in the field out the back of the practice, and sometimes in September or October in the early morning, if I'd slept at the practice that night looking after some patients, I went for a walk to clear my head before morning consultations and watched them locking antlers in rutting season. I always marvelled at how extraordinary it was that the antlers could be torn off or shed and then regrow, because antlers are in fact bone growing through skin. I came across a paper in 2006 written by Professor Gordon Blunn, Dr Catherine Pendegrass and Professor Allen Goodship at the Institute of Orthopaedics and Musculoskeletal Science of University College London, in which they had studied the interface between the antler and the skin and then recreated that using porous metal as a 'biomimetic' of this microstructure, so that they could potentially get skin to adhere to metal sticking through the leg of a human amputee. Their goal was to develop a bionic limb for a human. I wanted to develop bionic limbs for dogs.

Finally I got to meeting Professor Blunn and actually felt very much like a birdbrain as I sat outside his office waiting to be called into his tabernacle of power, thrilled and terrified that this deified luminary was taking the time to meet with me. His secretary Annie offered me a cup of tea and a gentle smile of encouragement as I sat there fidgeting nervously. As it turned out, there was no need for me to be nervous as he was a gentle, open, lovely man. He was the very first person who understood my proposal that vets and human surgeons should work together for the benefit of both animals and people, rather than just using the conventional model of an experimental animal – where a disease is given to an animal so that humans may benefit. My proposition was that he might allow me to use their technology to help dogs that really needed a new lower limb after a partial amputation, that I would fully inform potential clients regarding the options and, subject to their consent and ethical guidelines, I would work with his team to develop solutions, such that we would then share information for the greater good of my patients and his. He was more than happy to collaborate, and we have since become firm friends.

In 2007, surgeons at Stanmore Royal National Ortho-paedic Hospital fitted the first intraosseous transcutaneous amputation prosthesis (meaning that it went from inside the bone through the skin) on Kira Mason, who had lost her arm in the 7/7 terrorist bombings in London. That same year, with the assistance of Professor Blunn and a wonderful human plastic surgeon called Norbert Kang, I implanted the first ever bionic limb of this kind onto a Belgian shepherd dog called Storm who had a tumour which necessitated removal of his right front foot, as the family did not wish for him to have a full amputation of the limb. In both patients, human and animal, a rod was hammered down the marrow canal of the bone, attached to the base of which was a flange with pores, onto which the skin could be stitched, leaving a metal spigot sticking out (endoprosthesis), onto which a bionic limb (exoprosthesis) could be attached.

For the very first time, I was finally doing what I had dreamed of doing, helping an animal that needed help, and potentially preventing the deaths of animals that might otherwise be sacrificed to help humans, by sharing the knowledge side by side. The central goal of my life is to give animals a fair deal, in part by forging closer ties between human and animal medicine for the greater good, and I thought this was a breakthrough. But sadly, in the years ahead, the concept of a true two-way street of information was to prove much more difficult to establish than I had first imagined. I dreamed of One Medicine for all species, but at the time there were many people in both veterinary and human medicine who thought it was a birdbrained plan – and unfortunately there still are.

Soon afterwards, I operated on a second dog, Coal, to give him a bionic leg. Following an amputation to remove a tumour, his dad, Reg, became a good friend. Reg has worked in the security industry for many years and is a strong tough man, but around that dog he was marshmallow, and as I soon learned, one of the most kind human beings I've ever met. He wanted Coal's leg to be saved. Many in the veterinary profession considered that the operation should not be performed because most dogs do, in fact, manage very well indeed on three legs, and if they don't then they can be put to sleep. This remains how many vets still feel. That isn't how Reg and I felt.

I operated successfully and Coal made a full recovery. It was a great joy to me to see him performing one of his favourite tricks, which was to hold a drinks bottle between his two front feet, one of which was now bionic, and take the cap off the bottle with his teeth, whereupon he would assume the self-satisfied look of a very clever canine indeed, before he lapped up the contents. Coal ran around happily for fifteen months, but sadly was then put to sleep because of secondary cancer spread. Both Reg and I felt at peace then, and still do now, knowing we had done all we could for this magnificent dog.

Progress in human and veterinary medicine will happen anyway, with or without me; it'll just be slower if the professions don't work together. Human medicine is currently obliged by regulatory agencies for drugs and implants to use animal models, for very good reasons to ensure safety and efficacy, whilst animals that need those same solutions often cannot actually have them. Conversely, people see on *The Supervet* or when I lecture at academic meetings some procedures that they themselves cannot easily have yet. There is a self-evident mismatch. Currently a clinically viable platform for One Medicine does not exist.

Whatever the public or my profession think about me personally, I'd like to believe that I'm at least making people

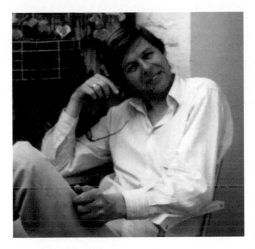

'Chase your dream – as long as you're doing the right thing – even when nobody is watching . . .'

'All you need is a reason big enough . . .'

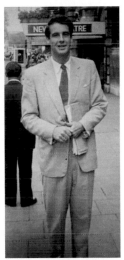

The inimitable Malcolm Drury (above) and Philip Gilbert (right) – my two great friends and mentors who believed in me, even when I didn't believe in myself. They inspired my 'field of dreams' and sustained me with encouragement and support at every turn. I look out from my office window at the cherry blossom and chestnut trees which I planted in their honour and miss them both very much every day.

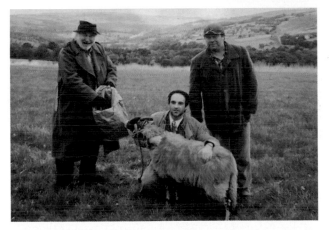

Thanks to Philip and Malcolm, I got to realise my secret dream of becoming an actor. Here I am on the set of *Heartbeat* with Bill Maynard (left) and David Lonsdale (right) – and a very pink sheep!

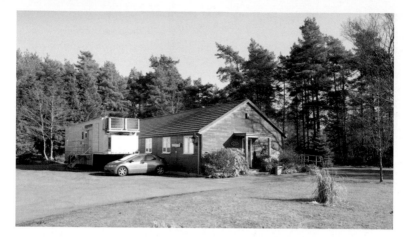

The hut in the woods near Tilford – with an MRI truck parked outside (above) – where Fitzpatrick Referrals took shape. I once scanned twenty-one animals and operated on nine patients in one weekend within those tiny four walls.

I ran out of money more than once during construction of the new site at Eashing (below), and at one point the builders were going to pull off site – but I knew I had to keep going to realise my dream of a state-of-the-art practice with extraordinary capability.

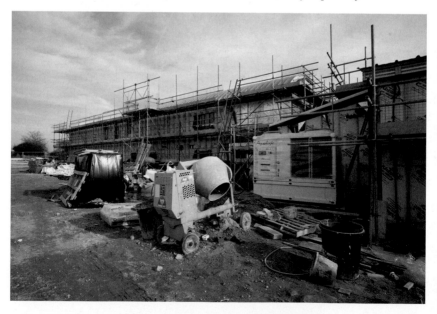

The old hay barn at the back of our farmhouse at home in Ballyfin, where Daddy inspired and educated me with his wise words (left). When I saw the old hay barn at Eashing some thirty years later, I knew in an instant that this would be my new home. Within the top corner of the old broken-down hay barn (right) I would build a beautiful lecture theatre in honour of Daddy where I could impart knowledge to the next generation too.

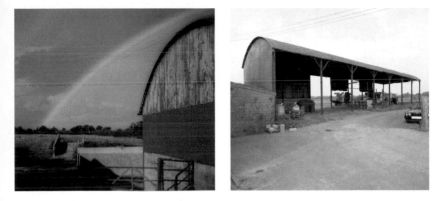

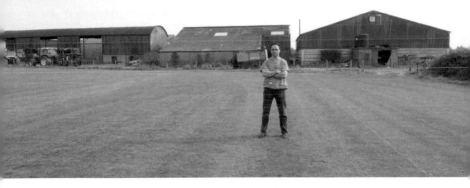

All of the effort was worth it to build my 'field of dreams' – the derelict farm in Eashing that would provide a home for Fitzpatrick Referrals Orthopaedics and Neurology Referral Center, where *The Supervet* has been filmed.

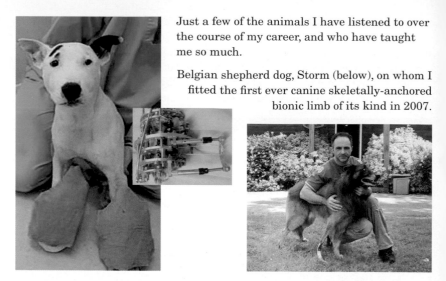

Just a few of the animals I have listened to over the course of my career, and who have taught me so much.

Belgian shepherd dog, Storm (below), on whom I fitted the first ever canine skeletally-anchored bionic limb of its kind in 2007.

Five-month old Staffy-cross, Winston (above), for whom I fashioned Wolverine-style claws after his horrific accident in 2005, and built a 'distraction-compression' external skeletal fixator (inset) that would allow me to transplant his tail vertebrae and parts of his pelvis to grow him new hands and wrists. The fishing line nylon in the picture is stretching the skin gradually to cover his sheared-off paw.

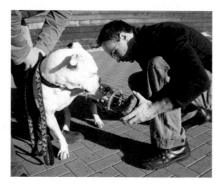

Following a partial limb amputation to remove a tumour, I implanted Coal (left) with a bionic leg. His dad Reg has since become a good friend. We are both very grateful to have had Coal's love in our lives. Both his and Storm's legacy is that other animals and humans will benefit from similar technology in the future.

German Shepherd Enzo (right) in the hydrotherapy pool with Chris Evans by his side. I shall remain forever grateful to that wilful, joyous, brave fluff-ball of wagging tail and gnawing teeth for introducing me to Chris, my greatest and most wise companion on life's journey.

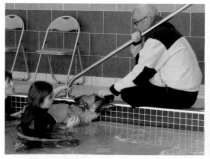

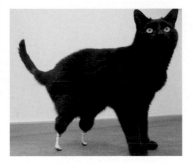

Oscar (left) with eight of his lives still intact. He was the first patient in the world, human or animal, to have two simultaneous skeletally-anchored bionic endoprostheses fitted, and that heralded a new era of possibility for both animal and man.

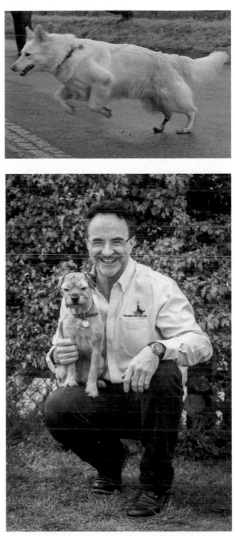

White German shepherd dog Mitzi (right), sprinting happily on her bionic leg in 2010. She would reignite my passion by helping me to rediscover the chestnut tree that I had planted for my dear friend Philip, and which I thought had died. Love and hope lived on.

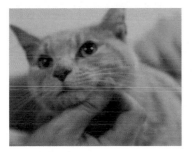

Tiger (above), whose life I quite literally held in my hands, when I restarted his heart, and who helped to open the door for the commissioning of *The Supervet*'s very first episode.

With Keira, my beloved Border terrier, the love of my life. She has been by my side every step of the way and not a day passes without her bringing a smile to my face.

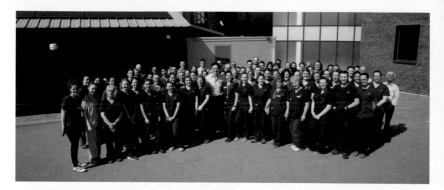

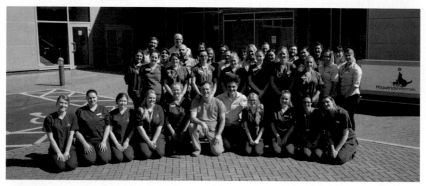

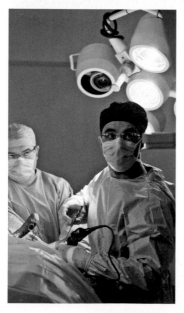

Avengers Assemble! My incredible colleagues in the Fitzpatrick Referrals Orthopaedics and Neurology Team – FRONT (top) – and Oncology and Soft Tissue Team – FROST (below). They are the extended Fitz-family, without whom none of what we do would be possible. I am incredibly proud to stand by their side, as we try every day to bring hope and healing into the world, for every animal entrusted to our care, and for those that love them.

Operating with my wonderful surgical resident Padraig Egan. He emailed me after watching *The Bionic Vet*, and I hired him a week later. He and others like him are the future of veterinary medicine and I am honoured to have played some small part in their education and inspiration.

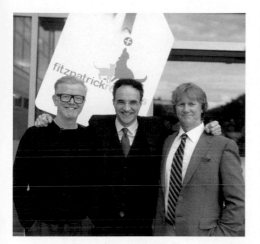

The opening of Fitzpatrick Referrals Oncology and Soft Tissue Centre, 2ⁿᵈ September 2015. I was grateful that my dear friend Chris Evans, who had helped to put us on the map with *The Bionic Vet*, cut the ribbon while standing beside another man, remarkably of the same name, Sir Professor Chris Evans. Sir Chris is a global luminary in human cancer research, with whom I hope to travel some of the road toward One Medicine.

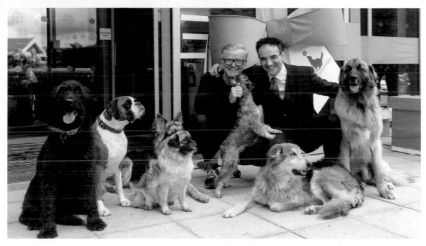

I was honoured to meet the Queen and explain bionic limbs and the potential for One Medicine to her, when she came to officially open the University of Surrey School of Veterinary Medicine in October 2015.

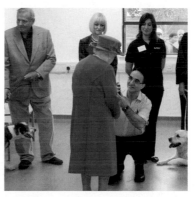

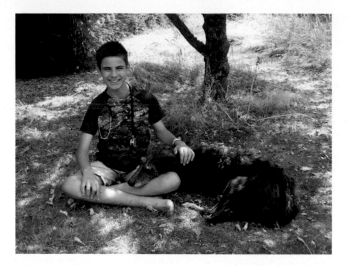

Lev wearing my stethoscope, with his beloved Willow by his side four years after the fateful night she broke her neck. If *The Supervet* inspires just one child like him to overcome adversity, and to follow their dreams, bringing light to the world, then it will all be worth it.

The double rainbow that appeared on the day I planted a cherry blossom for Malcolm right beside the chestnut tree I had planted for Philip. One rainbow is over the cherry blossom, the other over the chestnut tree – an incredible moment – my very own treasures at the ends of the rainbows, giving me love and hope every day of my life.

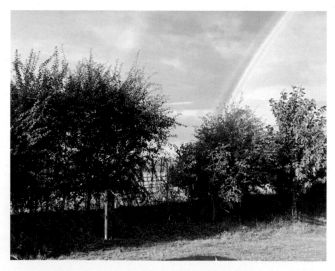

think. The important thing, in my view, is that this isn't about me; it's about whether these opinions are based on factually accurate information or biased isolationism, vested interest and intransigence. Public perception is changing, and increasingly the veterinary profession shall, in my opinion, need to change to keep pace with expectations and to uphold our good reputation. This should never be tarnished by untruths, monetisation or bias that is not evidence-based. We are a very small profession and I think it behoves all of us to listen to each other, to the animals and to the people who love them with respect – and if our opinions differ then let's discuss and debate openly and with integrity so that genuine and meaningful progress might be facilitated.

In that little hut in the woods in Tilford, my bionic journey began for me and for many animals which followed in the footsteps of Storm and Coal. This was a key stepping stone, not only towards my field of dreams – but also towards my life purpose.

From birdbrained beginnings, Fitzpatrick Referrals was about to take flight.

CHAPTER THIRTEEN

Winston and Wolverine

The Birth of Bionics and the Bank

Just as I moved to the hut in the woods near Tilford in late 2005, I saw a case that redefined my practice of veterinary medicine. The man was hunched up in anguish as he came into my consulting room, a small five-month-old white Staffy-cross puppy folded in his arms. Winston's front feet had gotten trapped under the wheel of a car and he had been dragged along the road. He'd suffered horrendous injuries to both of his front paws, losing one almost entirely. Nearly all of the wrist (carpus), palm (metacarpus), knuckles (metacarpo-phalangeal joints) and lower arm bone (radius), not to mention more than half of the skin and flesh, was gone on the right front paw, leaving only his fingertips. On the left leg, most of the wrist and the lower arm bone and a big chunk of flesh had also been shorn off. This wasn't a wait-and-see moment: this was do or die.

Winston was an integral member of this man's family and he asked if I could save him. I said I didn't know. '*It would be kinder to let him pass*', '*It isn't possible*', '*There is nothing we can do*' – I'd heard those words all my life and, indeed, had used them myself on many occasions. The puppy obviously couldn't be left to suffer in this manner and, because of the major tissue loss affecting both front legs, it was, indeed, reasonable to say that there was nothing that could be done and that it would be kinder to allow him to pass away peacefully. The question of whether to treat Winston or to put him down was by no means straightforward – his injuries were so severe that any procedure would be risky and costly and the outcome was uncertain.

No two situations are exactly the same and, of course, there absolutely are circumstances where a suffering animal should be put down. When faced with the choice to perform what may be complicated surgery requiring prolonged use of painkilling drugs, it's often very difficult to assess how much suffering the animal would have to endure, the life expectancy and the quality of that life and, in addition, what the odds for success are, at what cost and with what level of sacrifice by the family. Having said that, I believe that there is an ethical and moral line that, as veterinary surgeons and guardians of animals, we should never cross. Suffering for too long without good hope of a pain-free, functional quality of life remains the arbiter for most vets, including me. There remain challenges in defining what 'too long' means as a recovery period for an animal, and vets' opinions vary depending on their individual perspective. In cases of human medicine, meanwhile, the answer for the most part is 'as long as it needs to be'. Also, options for providing functional quality of life are improving all the time, so this subjective judgement is a moving target.

Between any vet and anyone who loves an injured animal, it is these criteria that determine where the line must be drawn – someone keeping an animal that is clearly suffering alive just because they can't bear to let go, for example, is understandably a very challenging situation for all concerned. Faced with a difficult decision, as in the case of Winston, I put it to my team and I now put it to you: imagine yourself in the position of any member of this family, imagine looking Winston in the eye and having to decide if you would 'turn out the lights' while knowing there was some chance of successful treatment available. Maybe you would; maybe you wouldn't. Like every veterinary professional, you are entitled to your opinion. I think you will agree that it's incredibly tough to call.

Our professional oath is this promise: 'Above all, that my constant endeavour will be to ensure the health and welfare of animals committed to my care.' This is a complex ethical landscape. In most cases concerning a child, we wouldn't baulk at the prospect of multiple surgical procedures over several years, if that is required in a complex trauma or limb deformity case: the life of a young person is understandably valued as greater than the life of a dog. I understand that and I respect that view, though I believe that we also need to consider the dog, Winston, for example, as a sentient being; a creature that has feelings, needs and wants that should be taken into account. Research has shown that dogs and cats can feel happy or sad, excited or disappointed, depressed or elated, and that these feelings may be similar to ours, even if they cannot express them in the same way that we do. If Winston could speak our language, he might be saying, *'It's just my front legs that are badly broken, can't you even try to fix me?'*

That's not anthropomorphism – I am a farmer's son, after all, and I do recognise the hierarchy of species; it's just that I'm sick of hearing, 'It's only a dog' or 'It's only a cat'. I signed up to be governed by the Royal College of Veterinary Surgeons, and I therefore see my primary vocation as looking after the welfare of animals, which is quite separate from the welfare of humans, all the while fully recognising and fully adhering to our governing body's clear stipulations that veterinary surgeons are also responsible with regard to the welfare of the guardians of the animal.

As stated in the RCVS guide of professional conduct:

Veterinary surgeons must be open and honest with
clients and respect their needs and requirements, must
provide independent and impartial advice and inform
a client of any conflict of interest, and must provide
appropriate information to clients about the practice,
including the costs of services and medicines, and
must communicate effectively with clients, including
in written and spoken English, and ensure informed
consent is obtained before treatments or procedures are
carried out.

In this context, I discussed fully all options, expected consequences and costs with Winston's dad. The family was going to need not only emotional resilience but also significant financial wherewithal to try to save his paws, but, in my view, they had the right to choose what best to do in their particular circumstances for their beloved young animal friend. This was long before *The Supervet* show, and the surgery that was needed for Winston was at the cutting edge for that era of veterinary practice in the UK. I was aware, therefore, that in performing this complex surgery, even if it were possible, I might be judged critically for 'pushing medicine too far', and that the family might also come under fire for saving Winston's paws at too high a financial cost.

Clearly no human doctor operating on a child would be questioned in this way if it were a privately funded operation, nor would the family be criticised for spending the money. The question I'm asking is this: from a rational point of view, notwithstanding the hierarchy of species, in the case of Winston, does society have the right to judge the amount of money that the family spent of their own volition? Furthermore, is it right that today some sectors of the media sensationalise the amount spent by any person on any animal, which they do regularly, often with regard to cases handled in my surgery? I agree that everyone has a right to their opinion, but do people have the right to criticise individuals for spending their own money on an animal, or to judge what is or isn't morally defensible?

I received such criticism back then and have heard it time and time again since – and I've grown tired of arguing the point, accepting that entrenched views rarely change even when confronted with sound reasoning and logic. Clearly there are governance issues which must be adhered to for the judgement of morals and ethics, but the fact that it remains fair game to criticise someone who spends money on a family companion animal, while someone who spends money on a material luxury item like a sports car, vintage champagne or designer shoes mainly goes without comment, or may even be praised, smacks of misplaced priorities in my opinion.

In Winston's case the fact of the matter was that unfortunately funding was very limited for any life-saving surgery. The family had young children and could only afford a relatively small contribution towards what would undoubtedly be an expensive undertaking. This remains the all-too-common challenge of veterinary medicine: the profound desire of the family and the vet to do everything possible to avoid the heartbreaking decision for euthanasia, versus the stark reality of affordability. In the UK at present, there is no national healthcare system for dogs or cats, nor is there elsewhere to my knowledge, and therefore any vet can be restricted in what may be possible depending on the circumstances presented. Animal charities which run veterinary practices through public donations do a fantastic job but necessarily have restrictions on the amount they can spend on any one case because they must look after the greater good of as many animals for as many means-tested people as possible.

There always have been, and still are, situations where there may in fact be nothing we can do and a decision may need to be made for euthanasia as the best option, but advances develop apace and the goalposts are constantly moving. Many times in the early nineties, I put patients to sleep that today I could potentially save and get them recovered in a reasonable timeframe. The challenge, however, is that some veterinary and public opinion may not have caught up with advances in possible techniques and technologies and this frequently results in me being accused of performing a particular technique because *I can*, rather than because *I should*. Of course, nothing could be further from the truth. To do such a thing would compromise my own ethical code, which is something I will never do. I have never picked up a scalpel blade if I wouldn't perform the same procedure on my own dog, Keira, whom I love very much. The fact is that nowadays we can very well control pain during postoperative recovery and I feel we should judge the recovery time duration (which for Winston would likely be quite long) in the light of overall life expectancy (which for Winston was also long). An entirely different set of judgements, in my view, may apply for a twelve-year-old dog with multiple limb issues and an anticipated life expectancy of one year.

I predict that many of the procedures performed in neuro-orthopaedics in dogs and cats that vets or members of the public may baulk at today will be commonplace twenty years from now. As Charlie Mayo said when he helped found the Mayo Clinic in the nineteenth century, 'the truth is ever-changing!' For example, where I grew up, performing a hip replacement on a dog would have been considered ridiculous beyond belief, and the same is obviously still true in some areas of the world. When I graduated total hip replacement remained rare, but now I have performed nearly a thousand such procedures. A hip replacement on a cat even today in the UK is considered exceptional, for no good reason in my opinion, since it's well established that although there are risks for any surgical procedure, simple or complex, the complication rate for standard total hip replacement in ex-perienced hands is low; recovery from this operation in dogs or cats is generally rapid and quality of life usually excellent. Furthermore, it's been scientifically shown that for most patients, total hip replacement is superior to the alternative of doing nothing or chopping the femoral head off (femoral head and neck excision). Sadly, some people are very quick to judge and very slow to try to understand. Even knee replace-ments in cats is now readily available and proven successful at my practice.

In Winston's case, I felt that something, although very challenging, might be possible. At that point, nothing that I knew of in the veterinary literature described a viable solution, and we didn't have bionic limb implants for dogs in 2005. I had to weigh up five key issues surrounding the potential procedure: amputating one leg, with the other so badly damaged, was a non-starter; a solution wasn't obvious as it had not been done before; even if it were possible the client couldn't afford the level of surgical intervention needed involving both front legs; Winston would have to go through an inevitable period of post-operative recovery; and lastly there would be significant risks and an uncertain outcome. This was a perfect storm, which would in many circumstances prompt a decision for euthanasia. For all of these reasons, even now, in the vast majority of veterinary practices, Winston would have been put to sleep. 'I'm sorry, there is nothing we can do' is a common conclusion when financial constraints alone are considered, never mind formidable medical challenges.

That statement is now often factually inaccurate, even though I genuinely believe that veterinary professionals are trying to do their best in any given circumstance. If a difficult surgical challenge is presented and in fact there is something that can be done, but the practice doesn't offer it, can't afford to perform it within the client's budget, or doesn't agree with it, for whatever reason, I question whether a veterinary surgeon has the right to definitively advise euthanasia without a thorough explanation of the rationale, since the client may have a different opinion when all options are clearly and transparently disclosed. The honest approach would be to say: 'I'm sorry but there isn't enough money to cover this procedure, there is a significant risk of failure, we do not at this practice or within this group of practices offer any solution for this problem, so it's up to you if you would like to have a referral elsewhere. You also need to be aware that your dog (or cat or rabbit ...) may have to go through a lot to get to the other side, so it may be better to allow him or her to pass away peacefully now.'

That's the truth.

Conversely, the statement 'there is nothing we can do' may, in fact, be the best thing a vet can say, because then people don't feel responsible or feel they haven't done their best. Over the years since that first case with Winston, I have also heard it said that, by providing too many options, I make things more difficult for families and also for the veterinary profession; and that I make people feel bad when they can't afford one of those options, or the aftercare is impractical for them or they just don't agree with my approach. I respect the right of everyone to make their own decisions, and clearly there are many wonderful referral practitioners other than me in the UK and elsewhere who can offer many and varied solutions, both in my field of neuro-orthopaedics and in others. However, I still feel that it is my duty to the family who loves an animal to lay out all of the options, all of the time. I strongly believe that the majority would prefer to be apprised of all the options, even if they ultimately decline them.

Winston's dad asked me: 'What would you do if he was your dog?' This is the most common question that I get asked, as is the case for many veterinary surgeons in practice. The essence of this query is that clients look to me for compassionate, as well as professional, guidance. They want to know that I care, that I am doing my best and that they can trust me to do what is right without any ulterior motive or agenda. However, this 'opinion' would vary enormously depending on which 'me' you ask – the one now, or the recently qualified vet at the beginning of my career. The same is likely true for any vet advising from the perspective of the experience in primary care or specialist referral practice he or she may have at that particular moment in time. The perception and experience of any individual is inevitably moulded by circumstance over time, as is awareness and availability of the technology at that point and in that geographic location.

I have always answered the question 'What would you do if he was your dog?' straight up, openly and frankly. However, recently I have learned that if a procedure isn't successful, sometimes the grief-stricken guardian of that patient might retrospectively feel that I have swayed their decision by stating 'that was what I would do if it were my dog'. In Winston's case, I might have said: 'As long as Winston doesn't suffer and we can control his pain with a reasonable chance of recovery, I will try my best to save him, but there isn't any technique published right now to do this and we'd have to think of something.'

I now answer that question of what I would do with the proviso that my governance indicates that I am not allowed to influence any client's decision and that all I can do is to tell the family truthfully that I never go into surgery unless I would perform that surgery on my own dog Keira in similar circumstances, and that while I hope to succeed, I am fallible and my clients need to be aware of the risks, which I then list. I emphasise that my job is to give them all of the options and that, while clients must make the decision for themselves, they are entitled to another opinion, if they so wish. In addition, I state that we always need to do the right thing for the patient and if suffering becomes evident then we may need to acquiesce to euthanasia. I reassure them that whatever their decision is, I shall hold their hand and do the right thing at all times.

'The right thing' for any patient is also a subjective judgement by clients, vets and insurers. Situations can arise where a clinician or insurer advises that a client should not have a

custom implant or prosthesis of any kind, even though techni-
cally all standard commercially available joint replacements
are in fact prostheses. If the particular implant system, such
as a customised joint replacement, isn't available universally,
I think it's important that clients have the freedom to seek
out where it is available, and still be able to work with their
primary care clinician and insurer to get the best possible
outcome for the animal they care about. I predict that we are
moving into an era where failure and success rates, including the actual indication for the procedure in the first place,
will need to be openly stated by clinicians and institutions.
Then 'value for money' can be assessed and compared per
condition and per technique either by self-paying individuals
or by insurers.

I recently compared the cases that constitute my operating list now to those that populated my daily list ten years
ago. Most of my cases nowadays are not routine, have already
seen several veterinary professionals, have not been offered
options or, for whatever reason, options have not been considered. Because technology moves quickly, if clinical need is
matched by implant availability I've tried to provide options
that hitherto haven't been available, and offer more than
thirty techniques or implant systems not currently available
anywhere else. This isn't self-aggrandisement; this is innovation because of frustration, and otherwise desolation if
limb or life can't be saved with conventional options.

On some occasions, it has even been implied that my
outcomes are 'dressed up' for the television show and that
my failure rate is high, so therefore clients should not seek
my opinion. The reality is that it's difficult for families and
broadcasters to show the stories of the animals for whom
treatments fail on television and I am forever grateful

to all those who allow failure or the death of their animal companion to be shown on *The Supervet*, because that's not easy. However, it is real life, and is shown as such without embellishment.

I strongly acknowledge that there is no surgical procedure, no implant system and no surgeon that succeeds all of the time. My own experience has been that commercially available implant systems fail as much as custom implants in my hands and that the more surgery of a particular kind I perform, the better I get and the lower my failure rate. However, as conditions previously deemed untreatable now have viable solutions, sometimes failure rates are unknown until surgery is actually performed. This is self-evident, but both clients and regulators have to recognise that. No amount of computer testing or dead-patient operating can truly predict real life. I have been categorical in my publications, lectures and in this book about the failure rates of the procedures I perform and this data is therefore in print when accrued. These include both commercially available and customised options. At the time of publication, I am scheduled to give six lectures at major international conferences in 2018 in which I shall speak purposefully and openly about failure and ethical responsibility, for which the abstract notes are available for any member of the profession to read for themselves.

For Winston back then, the bottom line was that if the family did not want him to be put to sleep, and even if I could have offered any solution, their financial wherewithal would not have covered all the costs incurred and therefore I would have had to give considerable time, effort and equipment for free, which ultimately the bank would pay for but they wouldn't like it.

Fitzpatrick Referrals remained in the converted hut

in the woods in Tilford as an interim measure while I was trying to pull enough financial resources together to build my new state-of-the-art practice on the farmland in Eashing. It was going to cost many millions to secure the location and build the facility. It's obvious that no financial lending institution expects a shopkeeper to give away a loaf of bread, and yet as a veterinary surgeon, because each case has deeply invested emotions, one would love to be in a position to offer every treatment or procedure less expensively. But with that approach, I would never have been able to build my dream buildings, with facilities of extraordinary capability, and that, ironically, would then have deprived a larger number of animals from receiving state-of-the-art care long term.

Nevertheless, at the time, I couldn't bear to put Winston to sleep, nor could the family, so we decided to try to save him. Initially, I just cleaned all of his wounds and built an external skeletal frame from aluminium rings with clamps, pins and wires that went into the bones above and below the damaged portions to suspend the defects like a spanning bridge, allowing the tissue, blood vessels and nerves to declare themselves dead or alive. Winston could walk on the bottom part of these frames, which transferred the ground load to the upper parts of his forearms and elbows. Over the following days, all dead tissue was removed and fortunately the blood and nerve supply to his front feet held up. On the right side, his lower arm, wrist and palm were absent, with the frame holding the toes onto the upper forearm, and on the left, most of his wrist and lower forearm were missing. There was also considerable tissue and skin loss. I needed a solution to fill the gaps in Winston's limbs.

First, I tried to use loose bone marrow graft harvested from the tops of both tibiae (shin bones), the bottoms of both femora (thigh bones), the tops of both humeri (upper arm bones) and the wing of the ilium (pelvic bone), but this loose graft, the harvesting of which is accepted practice, wasn't enough and didn't incorporate well because there wasn't enough scaffold structure or organised blood supply there to support the growth of new bone in Winston's paws, and the defects remained in the bone, and surrounding tissue and skin. I was running out of options.

Surgical innovation has been defined as: 'A new or modified surgical procedure that differs from currently accepted local practice, the outcomes of which have not been described and which may entail risk to the patient.' It has been proposed that such innovation is acceptable when there is a laboratory background to the research or the surgeon has spoken to other experts in the field, the institution has the field strength required to support the endeavour, and the institution has the stability and resources necessary to undertake such a surgery and to protect the patient as far as possible.

In regard to Winston, as has been the case for many of my innovations down through the years, I had hit a brick wall, and I was faced with a stark choice: I could either go ahead, without this advisory structure in place because it didn't exist at the time, and carry out innovative surgery, or I could put Winston to sleep. I thought of my childhood hero, Wolverine, and I reasoned that if I could fashion some rods like Wolverine had in his knuckles, then potentially I could thread bone blocks onto those rods and perhaps make them grow into new paws for Winston. Wolverine's claws were made from the fictional metal alloy adamantium, the imagined most indestructible metal ever synthesised on earth. Needless to say, even if I could somehow make this envisaged procedure a reality, rather more run-of-the-mill stainless steel claw rods would just have to suffice.

Far-fetched as this vision of Wolverine may seem, the original concept of filling bone defects using an external frame suspended on wires came from the Russian doctor Gavriil Abramovich Ilizarov by means of what he called 'compression-distraction'. In 1944, after graduating from medical school, Ilizarov was sent to Siberia to work in a small industrial town, Kurgan. The casualties from World War II were catastrophic and millions suffered from non-union fractures, chronic bone infections (osteomyelitis), deformity and large bone defects. With almost no antibiotics and no previous surgical or orthopaedic training, Ilizarov was faced with the inevitability of carrying out countless amputations on the wounded unless he could find a solution to salvage the limbs – a similar scenario to the one I faced with only one patient, Winston.

Ilizarov had seen rings attached to bone by metal wires and pins before, with adjacent rings attached together to stabilise bone for healing, but his big breakthrough was discovering how to move the rings relative to each other so that bone between the stabilised segments could be induced to actually grow by special cycles of 'pulling-apart' with specific rate and rhythm.

Ilizarov constructed two metal rings above the defect, attached with radial wires like the spokes of a bicycle wheel to the bone, and attached that apparatus to another two rings similarly mounted on wires below the defect. Then he used threaded rods that he turned so that the rings on either side of the defect moved apart to stimulate the bone cells to grow. He could then distract the rings gradually and fill the defect in a process called distraction osteogenesis. However, this was for a single long bone. In my case, Winston was missing four short bones in this palm, the metacarpals, so this technique wouldn't work on its own since the segments remaining were very small and incomplete due to shearing off, and the gap was massive.

For a long time, Ilizarov faced scepticism and resistance from the medical establishment in Moscow – allegedly, he made the wires from actual bicycle-wheel spokes and the rings for his frames from the gaskets of old tank engines from the war – but the results of his technique for the treatment of non-union fractures spoke for themselves. In 1968, he successfully operated on Valeriy Brumel, the 1964 Olympic champion, and a long-time world record holder in the men's high jump, who had injured his right leg in a motorcycle accident and over the three preceding years had apparently undergone seven invasive and twenty-five non-invasive surgeries. None were successful until Ilizarov's intervention. This procedure brought Ilizarov to the attention of the world, but especially America. Before his death, he trained a wonderful surgeon called Dror Paley, who travelled to Kurgan from Canada and who is now a globally recognised world leader in the field of limb deformities based in Florida. I learned how to apply such frames initially from Dan Lewis at the University of Florida veterinary school and later from Dror Paley himself, who has since become a great friend.

In his publications, Ilizarov had hinted at what I might be able to do for Winston – a technique that purported to somehow stabilise a recently harvested dead piece of bone and induce it to act as a scaffold and be incorporated into the skeleton by both compressing and distracting around it, as it remained stationary. This was a tall order – especially for four small bones of the palm, side by side, in a very compromised environment.

To do this, I needed to find multiple pieces of recently harvested and compatible dead bone with a cortex ring – the hard outer bit of a marrowbone – and somehow stabilise them in rows to reconstitute the metacarpal bones of Winston's palm. So I removed his tail and extracted the vertebrae, which were all small and round, just like the palm (metacarpal) bones of a paw. I now had six usable vertebrae, which were about the right length when stacked in pairs, end to end. This is where Wolverine's claws came in. I threaded each of the pairs of vertebrae longitudinally along each of three wires where the metacarpal bones should be. I still needed a fourth metacarpal bone and for this I removed the front of Winston's pelvis bone (ilium), cut it into two crabstick-shaped rectangular blocks and then stacked them in the same fashion.

I suspended these four longitudinal Wolverine wire claws onto a rigid arch at the level of the toe bones, right up against the knuckles (metacarpophalangeal joints), which had mostly been shorn off on the road. I linked this to another rigid ring above the wrist (carpus) and below the elbow. This stabilised the new bone segments. I then mounted further rings on wires like the spokes of a bicycle wheel above and below the wrist in between the stabilising rings and attached them together with three threaded rods with a special nut on each rod, allowing me to move this second set of two rings apart or together by a quarter or half a millimeter at a time. This was the 'compression-distraction' of dead pieces of bone that had been detached from their blood supply.

Using specific cycles (rate and rhythm) of distraction and compression, I hoped that blood supply would be attracted into the transplanted bone blocks, and further hoped, as research suggested, that this specific movement would create electrical charges called streaming biopotentials through the small 'canaliculi' channels of the bone. In this way, the mechanical strain pattern, which isn't too much or too little – called a mechanostat threshold – can theoretically stimulate certain biological molecules and ionic pathways in bone cells that could potentially induce incorporation of the tail verte-brae and the bits of the pelvis as a new series of metacarpal bones for Winston.

Thanks to Ilizarov and Wolverine my plan worked. The pieces of bone did in fact grow into a new palm for Winston. I shored up both wrists with more bone harvested from the pelvis and got them too to fuse together for both front feet. I used another arch mounted at right angles to the original apparatus on two threaded rods and nuts, which gradually pulled the skin across the defect, using fishing line as an anchor pulley and gel to keep the tissue moist.

Winston was such a beautiful puppy and a complete joy as a patient, always happy whenever he saw me, if not waggy-tailed by default. When he came in for adjustment of his frames or for X-ray pictures, he just shook his whole back end in eager anticipation of more cuddles from me and all of the team of nurses who looked after him through multiple procedures and five months of care. These were arduous surgeries and it was a long journey for both Winston and his family, but when he ran on the lawn outside the hut in the woods at the end of it, happy, pain-free and carefree, with his whole life ahead of him, we all knew it had been totally worth it. If I had failed, it might be said that we had 'put him through too much', but looking at him as he ran about, it seemed inconceivable that we might have turned out the lights on his life just five months earlier. He was without a tail – but certainly had a tale to tell!

Coincidentally, it took both Ilizarov and me twenty-three years to achieve specialist recognition, in my case a diploma in small animal orthopaedics and in his, a doctor of sciences. When I read his translated doctoral thesis, which helped to inform Winston's surgery, I could feel Ilizarov's pain in dealing with the cynics. Ilizarov suffered opposition from the Moscow medical establishment until the last years of his life. In 1991, just one year before his death, he was elected a full member of the Russian Academy of Sciences. Despite numerous awards and worldwide recognition, he was never elected to the USSR Academy of Medical Sciences. I guess a man is rarely a prophet in his homeland. He set up the Russian Ilizarov Scientific Center for Restorative Traumatology and Orthopaedics in 1971, which was his field of dreams. This, in no small way, inspired my own at Eashing.

Winston went on to live a happy and active life but I failed to get the academic paper documenting the technique I had used on him published. The reviewers rejected it as I didn't have enough scientific validation and the editor said, 'I'm sorry Noel, it seems that this isn't ready for prime time.' There was 'nothing he could do'. I actually could understand the point of view of the reviewers because in essence I couldn't examine a dead body or definitively prove anything of the proposed mechanisms for healing. I genuinely believe in the process of examinations and in the process of scientific publication. One cannot have veterinary medicine that is based on subjective opinion alone; it must be based on hard science, evidence, efficacy and ethics, all of which need to be appropriately peer-reviewed. However, all new knowledge will only ever get registered in the literature by performing the procedure in the first place and proving its validity. I feel that this warrants acknowledgement by society and by our regulatory bodies: if I hadn't tried to perform something that hadn't been published before, then Winston would almost certainly have been put to sleep.

Ilizarov died in July 1992, around the same time as I was moving to the UK from Ireland to discover my future. He was the father of a discovery that changed my life, in the sense that it inspired Winston's procedure. Winston's circumstances were the first to draw my focused attention to the implications of bionic regenerative innovation in the face of lack of finances – and gave me a profound insight into what would be required to innovate in the future.

I yearned to create a veterinary practice where super-specialists worked together for the greater good and where the finances were reinvested for real and tangible progress. The drive to build a practice where a new era of veterinary medicine might be possible was entirely my choice. I was determined to work hard and that money would not be the central goal, but rather a necessary oil to turn the wheels of a revolution that I wanted to start. I always wanted to be able to do the right thing for the animal and, while I knew I wouldn't be able to help everyone in financial crises, I wanted at least some clinical freedom to try. This wasn't then, and still isn't now, an easy concept to sell to any financial institution.

At Tilford, we were all working extraordinarily hard to make the move to the site at Eashing a reality. In 2005, I was operating many routine cases alongside a small team of fourteen, including nurses and support staff, and we had low overheads. Ironically, routine cases generate more money, more quickly than operating fewer numbers of complex cases with higher costs and overheads, which reduce profit margins and are less attractive for financial institutions. Every operation and intervention costs money, not just in terms of the time of the clinician, but also the wages of the nursing and ward staff, overheads on the facilities, operative drugs including anaesthesia, imaging such as scans or X-ray pictures, implants, disposables such as surgical drapes and sutures, bandages and aftercare drugs, for example – not forgetting an added 20 per cent VAT. In fact, often the fee for the surgeon's time is about one-fifth of most invoices. In Winston's case, if the billing had been charged appropriately it would have cost in excess of £20,000. For similar time, equipment, staff, overhead and drug costs in a human patient with comparable injuries, it might cost three or four times that amount.

I ran out of money more than once during the Eashing build, on one occasion almost scuppering the entire project. I remember being at rock bottom: the builders were going to pull off site and it wasn't even nearly finished. In the end, I had to phase the project, converting two of the four derelict buildings first, and then when I could borrow more money, a third building was converted, and all three joined together to form the core practice facility that exists today. During this period, I changed banks three times because the financial risk analysis frightened lenders, but I had to secure the loans or the project would never have happened. There were certainly moments during those three years when my will and conviction waned, and it seemed as if everywhere I looked there were brick walls of complication and obstruction, rather than the concrete brick walls I really wanted to see, raising my new practice from the ground.

I remember lying on my back in the field behind the practice and looking up at the stars much like I had done when I was a child and had lost my first lambs. Now I really needed to be braver and stronger than ever before. Exhausted, I put the earphones of my Walkman into my ears and flicked the switch on a brand-new CD. The song 'Clubfoot' from Kasabian blasted in my ears, and I thought to myself, if there was a melody that massive in the world I'd better get up and get back fighting. Many years later, Sergio Pizzorno, who co-wrote this epic anthem, became a lovely friend and for my fiftieth birthday gifted me the actual guitar on which he wrote their song 'Put Your Life on It'. I was absolutely prepared to put my life on it way back then, and still am today.

Every other week in Tilford a giant truck with an MRI scanner inside would turn up very late on a Friday night. I got it plugged into a transformer on the side of the building and on Saturday mornings we started scanning all the cases which had been booked in over the previous two weeks. The most scans we performed in a single day was twenty-one, and in that same weekend I operated on nine patients with the assistance of four great nurses. Most of these were dachshunds with disc problems. MRI changed my life because historically we had to inject dye around the spinal cord and take X-ray pictures (myelography) to see where a disc may have bulged (protrusion) or leaked (extrusion), causing compression on the spinal cord and inducing partial or complete paralysis of two or even four legs. Myelography was nowhere near as accurate as MRI scans. Now, I could obtain a scan with the crystal-clear information I needed in half an hour, and I was operating so many of these cases that my surgery times improved, with the average disc extrusion hemi-laminectomy surgery (cutting into the vertebral roofs to remove the disc material) taking fifteen minutes from initial incision to closure.

I consulted and operated on four to seven cases a day, and it was this effort that made possible the incarnation of Fitzpatrick Referrals at Eashing in 2008. We were available seven days a week, twenty-four hours a day, 365 days a year.

This would never have happened without the help of so many along the way, especially my loyal friend, extraordinarily compassionate clinician and amazingly talented surgeon Sarah Girling who joined Fitzpatrick Referrals in 2005 and remains by my side to this day.

I continued to discharge patients after midnight so that we could make space in our limited kennels for the following day. I recently saw a lady in my current practice in Eashing who jokingly berated me because she couldn't pick up her dog after midnight since I wasn't available – unlike a decade previously when I discharged another dog for her at 1 a.m. because I had no kennel space for the following day. She told me I was slacking. In her eyes, I had been more innovative a decade earlier!

The changing financial landscape of veterinary practice in the UK has affected how Fitzpatrick Referrals operates today. The relatively rapid corporatisation of veterinary medicine is a fact of life all over the world. It's interesting to explore what is already in the public domain in newspaper articles, but actually, little filters through to public consciousness. For example, it's estimated that up to half of all primary care veterinary practices across the UK are now owned by venture capital equity groups, although potential clients may not realise it, as in most cases the name of the local practice hasn't changed. Some of these groups own hundreds of primary care practices, most have centralised referral centres and some have pet crematoria, own-brand drugs, online pharmacies, laboratories, out-of-hours surgeries, locum agencies and both online and retail shops. Some even have very buoyant public share listings. This is true for both large animal practices such as equine and farm animal vets, and especially so for companion animal practices. To sustain this model, the rate of acquisition of primary care practices in the UK is rapid and, with high prices offered for practices, it's completely understandable why someone who has spent their life working very hard and for long hours would want to sell to the highest bidder and simultaneously divest the shackles of onerous management.

In North America, Mars Incorporated are now the largest pet nutrition and veterinary care provider in the world, with several brands of pet food and more than 2,000 veterinary practices nationwide. Recently, they made their first acquisition of one of the five largest groups of vet practices in the UK, with an undisclosed investment reputed to be the biggest ever seen in the veterinary sector. Investor appetite for the veterinary sector shows no sign of slowing, and share prices in these companies continue to grow. In 2016, the market value for pet care products in the UK (measured as part of Europe) reached around 5.2 billion euros and 44 per cent of people have a pet in their homes. So this is now big business.

The corporatisation of veterinary practice has inevitably influenced the choices offered to the guardians of animals, and such is the way of the world for many businesses globally. Most families understandably have no idea which specialist or referral option to choose anyway, except by personal recommendation from their primary care clinician or a friend, so they generally choose what is offered and what is local, though an increasing proportion are prepared to travel great distances for appropriate care. It's also true to say that many don't even know they have choice of clinician, cost structure or technique. To some extent the availability of information on the internet regarding procedures which may or may not be viable will influence choice, as will advertising, but fundamentally families want to know that both the primary care clinician and the referral specialist desperately care, and are motivated only by what they perceive as the best choice for their much-loved animal friend.

In the years between Winston and today, my personal caseload has changed dramatically from high-volume, less complex surgeries with greater profit margins to lower volume, more advanced surgeries with higher overheads and smaller profit margins. Nowadays, a growing number of the less complex cases are operated either within the referral hospital affiliated with the veterinary group of the primary care practice or by travelling surgeons hired to operate by primary care practices. The same is true in the United States. I absolutely believe that generally these surgeons do a great job and, of course, these referral centres also offer many options for more complex surgeries. They undoubtedly deliver great service and animal care, which may be comparable to that which my colleagues and I can deliver.

This changing financial landscape may be a positive development for animal care generally. However, in assessing the drivers for the change in my personal referral caseload, I have observed with some concern that independent referral practices cannot survive unless they maintain a bond of trust and service with primary care clinicians such that they can operate routine cases *in addition* to more advanced cases. Otherwise, the business model that allows advanced techniques to evolve is unsustainable and will not be supported by financial institutions.

The truth is that unless someone has significant financial resource or an excellent insurance policy, today operations like Winston's are very unlikely to happen. In primary care practice, the skill set, facilities, equipment and aftercare are generally not available, and in the current model of referral specialist practice someone needs to cover the bill somehow. It could possibly be performed within a university setting with a clinical research budget, but it's very difficult to achieve grant funding for such an endeavour without specific outcome measures. Furthermore, in many veterinary schools, the clinical education is outsourced to privately, or corporately, owned veterinary practices, such that it would be challenging to see large clinical case numbers within a vet school environment where such clinical research could flourish if funded appropriately.

This has had a knock-on effect on the procedures that can be offered, since development of any new technique costs a considerable amount of money in the first instance and needs to be refined over several years. I invested in a specific company, FitzBionics, to make the implants that provide solutions needed by the animals I regularly see in my consultation room, because evidence-based advances in bionic and regenerative technology require money. However, financial institutions and venture capital would prefer to fund high-volume, lower-cost procedures with high profit margins rather than taking a longer-term more strategic view. As overhead costs go up and wages rise, it's increasingly difficult to perform procedures for reduced costs or for free. Lending institutions understandably require a return on their investment.

As far as I can see, Winston's procedure, or any advanced veterinary surgical procedure, is not attractive to current business models or venture capital funding. Advancing techniques in small animal referral practice does not generate the same amount of revenue as performing routine surgeries. In a nutshell, if I personally operated on relatively straightforward orthopaedic and neurosurgical cases every day, I would make more money than by performing advanced surgical procedures, and my financiers would be much happier.

Nobody can afford to fund surgeries like Winston's every week and still pay wages, overheads and bank repayments. This restricts the rate of evolution of new and better techniques, since finances always come into play. Insurance companies are also necessarily tightening the options offered because what they can afford to pay out understandably has to be justified by the premiums they receive. In essence, someone needs to pay for the advance of veterinary medical techniques or we shall continue to have to say 'nothing can be done'.

During Easter 2008, we finally moved Fitzpatrick Referrals to the field of dreams in Eashing where *The Supervet* TV show is now filmed. From 2005, when we started in Tilford, we had grown to twenty-seven colleagues. We had all worked very hard and had raised several million pounds to service the growing debt of building the Eashing practice. Ironically, if I'd stuck it out in the hut in the woods for a few more years, I could have retired a millionaire. Instead, ten years later, the business employs 250 people, outgoings have increased, and overall borrowings in this time have been in excess of £12,000,000. I have so far repaid less than half of that and remain several million pounds in debt. I wouldn't have it any other way. Since I started with absolutely nothing, I cannot end up any further back than that, and I am more than satisfied to have created a place that isn't about the buildings or the 'asset', but rather about the people who fill the practice with love and hope for so many.

Money does not and never will concern me or in itself motivate me because we're doing the right thing for the animals and for those who love them. All is good – so long as I don't hear the bank manager tell me, 'I'm sorry, Noel. There is nothing we can do.'

CHAPTER FOURTEEN

Keira

Love in My Life

Keira is an eleven-year-old Border terrier and is the love of my life. She came into my world on 30 December 2007 when she was three months old. I had been longing for a canine friend to be by my side on the journey towards achieving the dream, but because I was busy working at Fitzpatrick Referrals in Tilford, and building our new practice at Eashing, there was one big snag: I often worked sixteen- or eighteen-hour days, seven days a week – consulting, operating, writing surgical reports, giving lectures and running the practice. I considered it unfair for me to have a dog in my life and not be able to take him or her for daily walks. The irony is not lost on me that my very vocation to save animals precluded me from having that kind of love in my own life.

Fortunately, my nurse, Amy, was also desperate to have a canine friend for her and her young son, Kyle. We were chatting in the operating theatre late one night and we joked that I had no time and she had no money, so we'd make perfect parents for a dog. We had both always wanted to have a Border terrier and I had recently treated one called Reg.

Knowing my penchant for the breed, three weeks later Reg's breeder emailed out of the blue asking if I would like the last puppy in a recent litter; it was a very happy coincidence, indeed.

I was operating on the day our puppy was due to be collected and so Amy drove up to Newcastle and brought Keira home to Tilford. It was a supremely special day, and I'm very grateful to Amy for her partnership in looking after Keira and allowing me to experience this uniquely special and unconditional love in my life. As I held that little fluffy ball of joy in my arms, I reflected on how my father may have felt when holding me for the first time. On reflection, I realise there is a certain symmetry here: like him, I had been unable to collect Keira on her first journey home, and on the day when I was being brought home as a baby, my daddy had also been busy operating, well, dehorning cattle to be precise. I do, of course, realise that there is an intrinsic difference between holding one's baby and me holding puppy Keira – but she is the very first living creature that I have parented, and that I will love and cherish for the rest of her life. For the first time, I'd become a daddy, and it opened all kinds of emotions from within me. I was quite overwhelmed.

The word 'parent' comes from the Latin verb *parire*, which means 'bring forth', and in my opinion, one of my greatest achievements on *The Supervet* hasn't been the surgery, it's been to persuade the production company and the broadcaster to allow me to consistently call the guardians of any animal 'parents' and 'family' rather than owners. I don't believe in 'ownership' of a sentient life – I think we undertake volitional guardianship and that this bringing forth can be one of the most rewarding and reciprocally loving relationships that a human being can ever experience.

With Keira and me, this is the absolute truth.

Keira is named after Keira Knightley, my vicarious love interest. I fell in love with this little brown-and-black, hairy munchkin, with big long eyelashes, from the first moment she scampered into my office and jumped into my arms, her tail wagging and her eyes full of life. Love at first sight – and love until the end of life, and beyond; but I don't want to ever think about that. Many people have said to me down the years that the death of their dog has been more traumatic than many human deaths in their family, and I completely understand that. Keira is my little pal, my confidante, my counsellor, my calm in the face of any storm, and my closest friend.

For Keira and me work is home, and home is work. I often live at the practice. Back in 2008 in Tilford I sometimes slept on a mattress on the floor, having finished surgery late and then needing to monitor some patients overnight, which often fell to me, because our staff numbers were small. Keira would be by my side in wake and in sleep back then, and still is to this day. Now I have a bed next to my office where I can rest, which is great since I don't lose time in travelling home after a late surgery followed by an early morning start. Keira has a nice snuggly bed beside me; the only problem now is that, as she gets older, she snores very loudly indeed, so I have to wear earplugs. She doesn't seem to mind my snoring, though, which is good. One night she managed to snaffle a brazil nut and spat it out beside my earplugs. I woke up, clearly having rummaged for the earplugs in the middle of the night, with an earplug in one ear and a brazil nut in the other. She likes to be close by me, and particularly likes clothes with my smell on, so I often have to look for pants or T-shirts curled up in a ball somewhere under or around the bed, where she's preferentially fallen asleep in their niffy cocoon instead of in her cushy bed. She has made me laugh many times in the morning, waking up with my T-shirt, or some other bit of clothing, on her head.

I rarely take holidays, and so most days Keira is with me at work. From the very beginning, she has always been a very quiet dog and doesn't bark much. She's the most wonderfully easy companion; she has a crazy few minutes, a nice walk and then loves to sleep, and snore, much like her daddy, who works ridiculous hours and then goes crazy for a few hours at a rock concert, sleeps and snores. Peas in a pod are we, and totally compatible. She sits at my feet while I write lectures and academic papers, and is sitting at my feet now as I write this chapter – gently snoring. When I am writing up surgical reports at the end of a long day in theatre, Keira is by my feet giving me solace, oblivious to whether the operations were successful or failures. Every time I operate, I know that my patient is someone else's Keira, and I never forget that. She's been by my side when I've studied for my specialist exams late into the night and her love has kept me going when I've felt tired and unable to go on, because I'm doing it for her and for everyone else's Keira too.

Licking my bearded chin and scouting for crumbs on the floor of the practice are her favourite pastimes. She especially loves the staff recreation room where there are crumbs galore, and, truth be told, she, like many dogs, is anyone's friend if you have food to give her. Fortunately for me, both Keira and Amy understand my paucity of work–life balance, and down the years it's worked out great. We are Keira's joint parents and she's been an integral member of two families, mine at the practice with her extended Fitz-family, and Amy and Kyle's at their house too.

The relationship I have with her is one of pure, unconditional love. She has allowed me to be the very best version of myself, and her company has helped to save me from myself whenever I feel lonely, sad, confused or inadequate. If I experience some major stress or turbulent crisis at work, when I come back into my office to a snoring hairy fluff-ball she brings me peace of mind. She puts things in perspective and reminds me why I continue to do what I do. Whenever I feel stressed or the world is driving me crazy, I hold her in my arms, rub my chin on her soft fur and give her a huge snuggle. She has given me far more than I have ever given her and I'm indescribably grateful. No matter how bad the day has been, when she looks in my eyes or licks my beard, my mood always lifts, and life immediately takes on a sunnier disposition. Not a day passes but she brings a smile to my face with her quirky little ways, her happy disposition and her insatiable appetite to show love and be loved. My life would be a significantly duller and darker place without her. No matter how sad life seems or how grumpy I'm feeling in a given moment, she lifts me up with her cheeky bum-waggle, and when I am walking with her in the lanes and fields near the practice or near my house, I feel freer, more alive and more at peace with the world.

Keira has also comforted me through the deaths of close friends and several failed relationships. I'm not being anthropomorphic; I'm just saying how I feel when I'm in her presence – and I know I feel calmer, more peaceful, more loved, more supported and have experienced more solidarity with Keira than I have sometimes with human relationships.

Don't get me wrong; certainly I have loved people in my lifetime, both in friendship and in romantic relationships, too. I have hurt and I have been hurt. I understand entirely that one can't compare a romantic relationship to the love of a dog. *But,* I respectfully submit that we have a lot to learn from those feelings we share with an animal: if we could transfer just a little bit of that kindness and generosity of spirit into our human relationships, I think the world would be a better place. In fact, everything I have ever striven to do – every operation, every academic paper, every lecture, every education and animal festival I've ever been involved with, and including this book – all of it has been in an effort to try to protect and project this compassion and trust between a human and an animal, which I see in my consulting room every day and which I experience with Keira. If I could bottle this love and spray this perfume around the world, I firmly believe we would be infinitely better off.

I'm not sure if it was my own particular perfume, or some other elements of my demeanour that prompted a recent enquiry as to the nature of my human interpersonal relationships by my young nephew, Dylan, during a recent visit home to Ireland. The entire family were sitting at dinner, when little Dylan piped up in a broad Irish accent, 'Uncle Noel, are you a homosexual?' This was fair enough, of course, since I don't get to go home that often and kids grow up fast, as do their perceptions! Contrary to his perception, I am heterosexual. I asked him what prompted his question, to which he replied that he had never seen me with a woman. Needless to say, this brought the busy banter to an abrupt halt. My sister Josephine was just about to censure her son when I interjected gently that maybe he might meet me with a woman on some other occasion.

In my teenage years, I was never much of a natural with the ladies: in fact, I remained a virgin until I was twenty-one. There were many reasons for this, but it was mainly ineptitude, along with a typically Irish Catholic childhood, full of sexual guilt and denial – as well as my self-imposed solitude of studying, of course. I desperately wanted to do the right thing by the Church and by my mother, and growing up at that time in Ballyfin there was a profound sense of taboo and shame around sex and even *thinking* about girls. It was discouraged by the Church and only spoken about in terms of being sinful. I'll never forget the roasting I got when my mother found me on the stairs at home looking at the page-three girls of the *Sunday World* newspaper.

I remember vividly when, with horror, I first saw the inside of a womb in Mr Murray's biology class at Ballyfin College when I was twelve, and being even more horrified when I heard what the town boys from Limerick, Cork, Dublin and Galway had seen and done. I had seen and done none of the things they bragged about. In my primary school, sex or anything to do with sex, had never ever even been whispered. I was clueless. On the first Friday of each month, I knelt down in confession, where we had to recount at least three sins for which to seek absolution, and one of those would invariably be: 'Bless me, Father, for I have sinned: I have had impure thoughts.'

The first non-imaginary female I had 'impure thoughts' about was the beautiful girl in the corner shop by the church in Mountmellick. I have no idea what her name was. I have no idea if she was even actually that beautiful, but in my head she was an Egyptian princess. I was fourteen and I never had the courage to do anything other than wait after mass until the queue at the till was at its longest before I joined it, just so I could spend more time in the shop, waiting in line, looking and smiling at her. The only words I ever said to her were, 'I would like this choc ice please', or something similar. She smiled back at me brightly enough to melt that ice cream – and me – most Sundays, for nearly two years.

I remained absolutely useless at talking to girls all the way through school, and indeed there was never any need to do so anyway, as I was usually studying or working on the farm, and never met any. So my sister Grace helped me out and set me up with a lovely girl for the leavers' ball at the end of secondary school, when I was seventeen. There I was in my suit, all dressed up and on a bus from Portlaoise to Dublin to a nightclub, a place I'd never been to in my entire life before, and it showed. I was a spare tool, totally inept at any kind of romantic conversation or conduct, and so in the end – and I really don't blame the poor girl – my date went off and romanced the best-looking guy there. I was left propping up a wall, watching them sway in a close embrace for the duration of New Order's 'Blue Monday'. In my head I was thinking, 'Oh my God, this song goes on forever.' It was the entire 12-inch remix, all seven minutes and twenty-nine seconds of it!

During my first year at veterinary school, when I was cycling thirty-three miles a day and practising karate, I made physical gains but certainly none of a romantic nature. I had zero game, and in any case, what with the cycling to and from college and the endless studying to get to grips with veterinary anatomy, I had zero time to acknowledge any form of female human anatomy or deliver any sort of game, even if I had had the chance. I was terrified of failing exams and so most nights I was curled up with my books. Truth be told, I was also terrified of girls. In second year, I was supposed to go on a date with a girl I had met down at a disco at the Lansdowne Road Rugby Club – when the DJ was playing the Housemartins' 'Caravan of Love' – but I couldn't go because

I crashed my bicycle into a car and had my arm in a sling. I had no phone number for her, it being the days before mobile phones; she thought I stood her up and that was that – no caravan of love for me.

When I was nineteen and working in the hotel outside Philadelphia, I noticed a very attractive girl who came to lunch on a few consecutive Sundays. Her name was Judy, which I only knew because Matt, the suave lothario waiter, could get the attention and the name of any woman. I eventually plucked up the courage to make an excuse to get her coat at the end of lunch. Dry mouth, heart pounding, I asked in the most pathetic tone if maybe she'd like to go for a walk sometime. Go for a walk? What was I thinking? Doh! Complete doofus! She just smiled and said, 'I don't think so, but thank you very much,' and I went back with my tail between my legs to endure a complete roasting from Matt and the other guys at the bar.

I got a reprieve, though, because the following week George Benson was playing a few concerts at a venue next door and one of his guitarists came in and was sitting at the bar in the hotel while I was washing up the glasses. We got talking and he had a good listening ear. I told him my woes and of my attempt to ask Judy out, and he must have taken pity on me because the next night he came in he brought me two front-row tickets for the show – and lo and behold, when I took my life in my hands and asked Judy out again, after initial hesitation, she said yes. It was amazing – my first concert with a girl! I was so fired up that I might just have burst into flames. Unfortunately, my game was less lusty than my ardour, though, and when she dropped me back to the house I was staying at in her car, there was the awkward good-night moment where my lunging attempt at a kiss turned into a kind of cringe hug. You know the type where someone is patting you on the back saying, 'All right, it's time to let go now, you're squeezing the life out of me!' So we parted ways. (To this day, I hate it when I hug anyone and they pat me on the back, and I hug a LOT of people; in fact, most of my clients, every day. So let that be a lesson to you: if you are ever offered the Fitz-hug – No Patting!)

I did see Judy again and, against all the odds, we did eventually have a sort of a proper kiss. She came with me to a George Michael concert towards the end of my second summer in Philadelphia in 1988. He opened with 'I Want Your Sex'. I'm pretty sure we just looked at each other and kind of smiled with embarrassment. None of those shenanigans ever went on in my life until much, much later; I think both of us were well wired to Catholic guilt. (Strangely, on the very same day as I write about my date with Judy, George Michael has died, aged fifty-three. I really loved his music and I'm really sad he's gone. It's a little reminder that none of us are going to be around forever, so best just say what you have to say, and like my mammy and my dog Keira, love generously, forgive easily, and get on with living.)

In my third year at university in Dublin, the tiny one-room bedsit I shared with the Weetabix-thieving rat was no place to entertain a lady, even if I had been, in any way, shape or form, lucky enough to find someone remotely interested in me. But I did have 'my eye on' a girl. I thought it would be a brilliantly romantic gesture to pick daffodils on my way home from a night's work at the horse foaling facility where I was seeing practice, and take them to her before breakfast at her nice, big, redbrick house in the affluent part of Ranelagh. Sadly, I had no means with which to carry these flowers except inside my motorbike jacket, which I duly did.

I turned up at her house after a night of foaling, smelling of horse shite and, as she opened the door, I produced the big bunch of crushed daffodils from inside my jacket. She took one disdainful look at me, shook her head and closed the door again.

Later in my fourth year of vet school, however, things took a turn for the better when I met my first proper girlfriend at Jeanine's flat, above mine in Pembroke Road. She shall remain nameless for reasons that will become clear. When I say 'proper', a more accurate description in fact would be transient and misconstrued. I think I've always been an eternal romantic and, at that time, I was also considerably more gullible than most guys. I had a late start and an inauspicious beginning, so when, as a twenty-one-year-old, I finally lost my virginity after a spontaneous climb up onto the roof on a very sunny day, which in itself was a rarity in Dublin, it wasn't that wonderful – a lot of fumbling and rustling. At the time, I wondered why everyone had told me it was so great – but most likely it was just that I wasn't so great. When she went home to America, I saved up a few hundred pounds and sent that to her for a ticket to come back to visit me but she didn't show up. To this day, I'm pretty sure that she went to see her other boyfriend in France instead! Not a great start to my romantic journey, let's say. I was gutted.

I met my first really proper girlfriend, Helena, in the offices of the Ross Tallon modelling agency during my brief stint as a model when I was in my final year at vet school. I was sitting in reception waiting for a casting meeting when I saw this stunning girl with long blonde hair waft past, her perfume lingering, a redolent symphony of scent that I can still remember to this day. I had absolutely no idea who she was.

Luckily though, everyone had left the office momentarily and, quick as a flash, I flicked through the book of headshots on the desk. Her name was Helena – brilliant – and better still, there was her phone number. I heard voices from the next room and it was clear they were coming back imminently. Pen, pen; I needed a frigging pen! No pen to be found anywhere – but there was a screwdriver (I have no idea why) – so I literally scraped Helena's number onto the cardboard of a cigarette packet I grabbed from a bin and hoped to God I would be able to decipher it later.

I could and I did. When I called, her mum came to the phone and a nicer woman you couldn't find. I have absolutely no clue what I said except 'hello', but I must have fared better with Helena when her mum put her on because I bagged a lovely date with a lovely girl. That first meeting involved her coming with me to see a Great Dane called Thor at the small animal hospital of the vet school, followed by tea and sparkly 7up at Jurys Hotel in Ballsbridge. I was nervous as hell, but it must have gone well because soon we were a couple. Helena and I were together throughout most of my time as a large animal vet in rural Ireland. God bless her, she would turn up on a green bus from Dublin or on a train to the back arse of nowhere where I was living and working – usually with a bag of sandwiches from the café where she worked.

Helena and I would head out on farm animal calls together at one or other of the large animal practices where I worked after graduating from vet school. On more than one occasion this poor girl, born and raised in the city, was up to her knees in muck, or up to her elbows in blood, helping me with lambing or calving, or holding a torch in the freezing winter, with her hands shaking, numb with the cold. One of my most vivid memories of this time together was during an outbreak of redwater, a life-threatening cattle disease, common in marshy bogland – and bogland was the predominant land type surrounding the practice where I worked in Ireland at that time.

Redwater is caused by a bug called *Babesia divergens* and is transmitted by ticks. Basically the bug causes the red blood cells in cattle to explode, one after another, until the haemoglobin passes into the urine where it causes toxicity in the kidneys. The blood can't carry enough oxygen and the cattle basically bleed to death through their urine. By the time we'd be called to a redwater case, there might be twenty cattle lying dying in a field. It's a brutal disease and one has to act fast to administer a transfusion of blood from healthy cattle to the affected ones. Healthy cattle were lined up in a crush with a gate at the end upon which there was a ratchet that locked the head and neck of the first animal – easier said than done! All available farmhands were roped in, and each beast was held by the nose with tongs while I took a gallon-and-a-half or so of blood from the jugular vein, which was mixed in a bucket with a few spoons of sodium citrate to stop it clotting. This was then transported quickly by tractor, which carried several buckets in an attached transport box, to arrive at the fallen bovine soldiers. Then and there I transfused the blood into each of the forlorn beasts.

My vivid memory is of Helena, a girl from the heart of Dublin, standing in the middle of a bog in the depths of County Offaly, with her arms aloft in the drizzly rain, holding a big upturned plastic Lucozade bottle with the bottom cut off, which was acting as a funnel attached to a long rubber tube that filtered the cows' blood down into a needle inserted into the jugular vein of the stricken beast on the ground. Usually the cattle were so paralytic that keeping them still was no bother – but my God was it hard sometimes to get veins because the poor beasts were so bled out. Still, that was little trouble for me by comparison with poor Helena, who just stood there petrified, as blood trickled down from the wobbling crucible of the Lucozade bottle into her armpits. Fortunately, she was an incredibly resilient and determined girl, and the most wonderful help on that awful evening, where in the end, to treat all the cattle affected, we worked into the night by the lights of the tractor. After the transfusion I gave each of the cattle a drug called Imidocarb to kill the *Babesia* and this process was so successful that shortly thereafter many got to their feet and, though unsteady at first, walked off, as if some kind of miracle had just happened. But I wasn't a miracle worker – and Helena certainly had no misconceptions on that score.

Helena was and still is an amazing girl; beautiful, kind, and with huge integrity. I think she knew that the only way to be close to me was to travel alongside me. We went on many farm calls together in my rusty old yellow Mazda and we'd chat endlessly between calls, in all weathers, as we sped along windy country lanes. One day my trusty Mazda got stuck in a muddy lane and I got out to push the car backwards from the front. Helena didn't know how to drive, and as the car started to get some traction, she floored the accelerator, ripping the rusty exhaust off in the process. The car stood by us, though, day and night, its bonnet serving as a table for a Chinese takeaway one night, parked up at the side of a lake, on our way home after I had performed a postmortem on a cow. As we did that night, we often looked up at the stars in the sky and acknowledged how lucky we were. She was the first girl with whom I properly shared my life.

Once we spent the night at a farmhouse bed and breakfast

when we went to see a Prince concert in 1990 in Cork. We were lying in the dark in a very small bed when suddenly the door opened and a small child with no pyjama bottoms on wandered in and said, 'Mister, what are you doing in my bed – and have you seen my potty?' It wasn't a B&B at all, just a farmer turning his child out of his room to make a few quid. We rolled with laughter.

I was very lucky to have this relationship with Helena and if I had married her, my life would have turned out very differently. I would not have had my heart broken and I would not have broken any hearts. Helena and I split up for lots of reasons, but mainly because I wanted to move to London to follow my dreams. I could and should have explained it better to her, and I hurt her by leaving, which I was very upset about too. Sometime later, I was sitting in Heathrow airport thinking about her, the earphones of my cassette Walkman in, listening to Take That's 'Back for Good'. As the music washed over my aching thoughts, I did, indeed, have a picture of her beside me – and her lipstick mark was indeed still on a coffee cup sitting on the draining board of a kitchen I'd left behind. In chasing my dreams, I left Helena behind too.

I didn't realise when I was in farm animal practice that in many eyes, except my own, I was apparently the most eligible bachelor in town. Julia was the daughter of a client – at a guess in her early thirties – with a grand mop of tousled brown hair. She lived with her mother in a thatched cottage, of which, thankfully, I only ever got to see the kitchen, where there were two small piglets being bottle-fed, a lamb in a box on the turf-fired range and the Sacred Heart of Jesus lamp barely glimmering over the half-door through the smog from her mother's pipe.

As I trudged through the potholes, Julia's mother leaned over the half-door of the cottage, took the pipe out of her tombstoned mouth and spat a large chunk of phlegm and tobacco on the slurry-covered yard.

'There ya go now, late as ya like as usual!' she chided.

'Yeah,' I thought, 'I'm frigging knackered – this is my fifth calving today and it's barely afternoon.'

With one front leg and the head forward, and just one front leg down in front of the pelvis, it looked like an easy calving – and so it was. I just popped the head and first leg back in a bit and up popped the second leg. Then I propped the calving jack up on the cow's arse and got a rope around both front knuckles of the calf, followed by a rope round the back of the head below the ears and into the mouth, with each rope then attached onto one of three hooks of the jack. The saddle of the jack squeezed against the cow beneath the vagina, and then, crank, crank, crank on the handle, a couple of waggles of the jack, and out she came, quick as a flash. The calf landed squarely on the yard, I sat her up and pummelled the chest and head a bit as was normally done, and then her mother whipped round to lick the mucus. I whirled round too triumphantly.

And there she was – Julia, with a glint in her eye, standing holding a bucket of water and a bar of Palmolive soap. Now, I specifically say Palmolive soap because that's green and it had a little leaf engraved on the bar. After the death of the man of the house, Julia and her mother had been the recipients of one thatched cottage, one rather derelict farmyard, twenty-six cows, one Massey Ferguson tractor – with a roll bar for added protection – and one four-sod plough. So, all in all, quite a dowry, had I been thinking that way – which I absolutely assure you, I most certainly was not. It appeared that her father may have also bequeathed her one solitary bar of Palmolive soap, because I swear to God each time I went out to calve a cow, that bar of soap in Julia's hand got smaller, but the leaf remained – which led me to conclude that Julia sought my approval so much that she wanted to make the old bar look new again by re-stencilling the leaf on the soap for each visit.

Anyway, there she was holding a bucket full of steaming water in one hand, a bar of 'fresh' Palmolive soap in the other, a towel over her arm, which only had a few holes in it, and a huge grin under her freshly combed tousled mane. At this point her mother again pulled the pipe out of her mouth as if to say something profound, but paused, as though for dramatic effect. She wiped her nose with the sleeve of her coat, leaned on the roof of my rusty yellow Mazda and uttered the following immortal words which I shall never forget: 'There ya are now. Sure, my daughter Julia was thinkin' that her boots would look woeful well under your bed!'

I blushed in embarrassment, mumbled that I was already spoken for and that I was very flattered, while simultaneously handing her injections for a calf with diarrhoea. Julia and her mother were rural, good-living people, surviving as well as they could and sustaining themselves on their small farm without the help of a man. It was only years later that I realised how seriously flattered I should have been that these two women considered me worthy of sharing with them all their worldly possessions.

I suppose I could have got married a few times in my life, and in fact why I'm not married at age fifty seems to fascinate people more than anything else about me. It could be said that I gravitate towards animals, like Pirate in my childhood and Keira in my adult years, because I find human relationships difficult. The bottom line is that from my part-ners' point of view, I have been selfish – something that I have been told time and time again in no uncertain terms. So, for example, while I have been fixing a dog, a girl I loved has been in bed with someone else. That's a bitter pill to swallow – and yet I can see it from her point of view. Why should she put up with always being second best to a dog or a cat in crisis? She also has needs, dreams, hopes and aspirations – and they're not being served by me operating at midnight on a Friday, Saturday or Sunday night. That's a tough call – and nobody's really to blame here, but it doesn't hurt any the less. Yet, there are many other professions where people have to work long hours, like members of the armed forces, but I suppose that they also have extended periods of availability. I don't, but I have chosen my destiny with my eyes wide open and take full responsibility.

I should add that I have not been a saint either, so I can-not throw stones. I have had my fair share of relationships, haven't been as romantically tactful as I should have been, and have done foolish things. Sometimes life isn't simple, but hopefully the older I get, the wiser I become in that department. I'm quite sure that if folks were honest, most people have had failed relationships and may not be proud of how things have been handled once or twice in life, and so it has been for me too.

I can dress up the altruistic aspect of looking after animals all I like, but at the end of the day, there are only so many times that anyone can put up with not feeling top priority, regardless of the reason or how potentially noble it may be. The reality is that if one is in a relationship that's supposed to be mutually supportive, one's very being is undermined if there's always something more important than the other person in that relationship. It's a fair point, and as a dear friend once said to me, 'You don't deserve success in love, because you haven't put in the effort. If you put a fraction of the effort that you put into saving animals, you'd have the best relationship on the planet.'

The irony isn't lost on me that I spend my life looking after one animal after another, who are someone else's love, and have neglected my own. We all have our demons and unless I'm prepared to face mine and be willing somehow to balance my professional life with some kind of personal life, I have no right to expect anyone else to dedicate themselves to me or to align with my vocation. Any partner I may be with has a right to make her decisions too, as another close friend was wont to tell me, but I do actually feel that you can make someone the centre of your world, as part of a bigger universe that hopefully both of you want to travel through side by side. The universe I am aiming for is a new world order of respect for animals and humans side by side, through medicine and love, and that is reflected in what I first felt for my childhood dog Pirate and in what I feel for Keira.

I have battled with periods of profound depression and feelings of worthlessness throughout my life. There have been times when I have wanted just to check out. I have made bad mistakes myself, though I have genuinely had deep feelings for everyone I have ever held in my arms. Whether I messed up or they did, or we both did, I still care about them and, in some cases, I still very much love them. I can honestly say that the pain of love rejected is a hundred times worse than any pain I have ever felt. Worse than the pain of failure, or exams or worry about millions of pounds of debt: none of it even comes close to the pain of lost love. It's crazy that our brains, in all of their complexity, choose to fire these neurones repeatedly that can most hurt us, and very little of it can be rationalised – just the same old movie of pain playing over and over in my mind.

It's tempting to sublimate pain, or to not take personal responsibility, by saving animal lives, and I have been guilty of that, because there's always a life to save. It's much harder to slow the movie down, and to take a good long hard look at myself in the mirror. Truth be told, sitting down to write this book has been a self-imposed solitude and time of reflection that I have never, in my entire life, afforded myself. Being forced to look back on my life has been intensely painful, but also cathartic, and has brought some difficult truths home to roost that I had subconsciously or consciously avoided by working all the time. This, I think, is a good thing, and will hopefully reap dividends that far transcend these pages.

One thing I know for sure is that although my love for animals has taken me away from personal relationships, that same love for the animals has saved me too. Through their eyes I can see that my work really does matter, in spite of the challenges and heartache. When I reunite an animal that I have saved with the person who loves that animal, the palpable joy in the room soothes the acute pain of love lost that I may have experienced because of my work. Yet the dull ache remains, and I truly wish that I might have balanced the scales of life better – although without the solace of the unconditional love that Keira and other animals have brought into my life, I would have lost the very essence of why I exist at all.

On a more humorous note, I definitely do not have as active a romantic life as people would like to make out, and I can assure you that my romantic prowess is nothing like the rumours I have heard! These gossips have way too much time on their hands and some of their fabrications are quite elaborate. In fact, I wish I had that much time on my hands to be romantic.

Down through the years, both before and after *The Supervet* was aired, I have had some wonderful moments of amorous intent, and I have also received quite a few interesting gift items in the post: a pillow with a cinema ticket embroidered on it saying 'admits two' was kind of sweet. A picture of just a very short tennis skirt along with a tennis ball wrapped in a bow, accompanied by a note saying 'the ball's in your court, baby' – from a lady client – was certainly original.

I have had some fantastic relationships in my life, and I am grateful for every minute that someone I loved has spent with me. I have been so lucky in many ways, but at the time of writing I have no plans to get married – despite a hilarious line of enquiry by a tabloid recently. I gave an interview where they asked me the most romantic thing I'd ever done and I answered innocently, 'Planned the location of a proposal, which hasn't happened yet.' This is, of course, entirely true in that I know where I'd love to propose, but despite their inferences, it hasn't happened.

It's hardly surprising that I have met many of the people I have dated through my work, because that's where I spend the vast majority of my life. While still working at Hunters Lodge veterinary practice I started dating Tracy, the ex-wife of comedian Jim Davidson. She brought in her young daughter, Elsie, and her cat to my consulting room and I soon ended up loving all three of them, along with her two boys, Fred and Charlie. For four years I read them bedtime stories, watched *Blackadder* on repeat, played Pokémon and made up games with them. It was long before the TV show and I was quite naive about the media, until a journalist just walked into a consultation I was having with a couple and their dog, and shoved a tape recorder in my face. It wasn't far to throw him into the garden, fortunately. I was also lambasted in the press for wearing Jim's swimming trunks. I'm an awful swimmer, having grown up in the middle of Ireland with no sea or lake and learning to swim in a pool, like most other things other than looking after sheep, was far from a priority. So I didn't have any swimming trunks and Tracy gave me some. I actually didn't question where they'd come from, but I should have known. He wasn't happy and let the press know about it. Fair enough, actually; I wouldn't have liked that either.

Tracy was a great partner, but I can see that I was less than a perfect prospect: not only did I not own my own swimming trunks but I didn't have much time or money. On a weekend away in Rome together, I managed to give all our Italian lira to a taxi driver because I mixed up a few decimal points. Tracy was understandably furious with me and 'accidentally' locked me out on the balcony of our hotel room for a while. In the end, we went our separate ways mainly because my time was spent working as a vet or an actor, rather than with her. She needed and deserved more commitment. Wonderfully, though, Fred and Elsie recently came to my fiftieth birthday party and I was in awe that the little girl on the edge of whose bed I used to make up stories about magic vegetables and unicorns had just got engaged to be married.

I dated the singer-songwriter Cathy Dennis in the early 2000s. We met because of her lovely Labrador, Charlie, who in spite of my best efforts remained paralysed on his back legs after a spinal injury. Cathy was kind and lovely to me but it was a similar story in that my working schedule eventually drove us apart. How could it not? She'd come back from re-cording an incredible world-shattering song and I would be operating until 2 a.m. We both had to make a choice, and we did. I know that she would have wanted me to go on loving the animals as best I could, even if that took me away from her.

I sometimes wonder if there are strands of our relation-ship running through the lyrics of any of the amazing songs that Cathy has written. I doubt it, and certainly hope not with 'Toxic', or 'Sweet Dreams My LA Ex', although I wish that the Clay Aiken album *Measure of a Man* has some echo of me in there somewhere. The title song came out around the time of our break-up in 2003, and I had gone to The Ohio State University to learn from people who became some of my greatest mentors. I was nursing a broken heart, miser-able as sin, and walked head stooped, shoulders hunched through a Target superstore, utterly pissed off with life. I rounded a corner in this dishevelled state and walked right into a giant cardboard cut-out of Clay Aiken, with all of his CDs perfectly arranged in a rack beneath. I fell right over, on top of poor Clay and his beautifully manicured CD rack. There I was, on my back, surrounded by copies of *Measure of a Man* and a crumpled cardboard Clay Aiken, looking up at the giant metal-caged ceiling above and crying. Luckily the folks around thought it was just because I'd hurt myself, when inside it was just ironically pitiful to be felled by this particular CD rack.

Cathy and I remain good friends, and I'm sad that I didn't and couldn't give her, or in fact anyone else, what is needed in a healthy relationship. Mostly it's difficult to ask the ques-tions that circle my mind over lost love, and probably safer to stick with the aphorism that 'everything happens for a reason', whether I believe it or not. *'The world breaks everyone and afterward many are strong at the broken places.'* Ah, now here's the thing – in biology – the cross-linkage of collagen molecules in a non-anisotropic alignment is, in fact, commonly weaker than the original crimp pattern and when exercised may therefore tear again. Now that's where biology messes up Hemingway! I think I'm probably still weaker in the places I've been broken.

The irony of all of it is that I still love *love*. It cannot be bought and cannot be sold. It is more valuable than any other emotion or any material possession on the planet. It is indefinable, ethereal, ineffable and eternal. In fact, it cannot be defined; it can only be felt. The best attempt I have seen to define love in terms of the rational world is the movie *Interstellar* by Christopher Nolan. In it, an astronaut is displaced by time and space from the family he loves and he is beating on the back of a bookcase from which dust is falling into the real world a couple of hundred years and an ocean of space away. Behind him is a complex computer-generated algorithm of everything ever rationalised as dimensions by mankind. For me, of course, the point is that everything that we can rationalise simply cannot hold or define love. It's futile and it's impossible, because it is the thing that 'has no name', as Oscar Wilde once put it. And yet, because I'm an eternal romantic and a perfectionist, I have tried to rationalise love many times in my life. I have, however, discovered that neither romance nor perfectionism have anything at all to do with love.

A few years ago, I was driving home to Ireland with Keira by my side. We stopped by the roadside for a pee somewhere in Snowdonia in Wales. She licked my face and then was delighted to see sheep in the distance. As she stretched her legs, I huddled by the remains of an old tumbledown cottage in the bleating cold wind and drizzle. As I sat and watched Keira sniffing the air and exploring her surroundings, I began to cry. A serious relationship had ended not long before, my heart was broken and I had been unable to patch the cracks. I still loved but that love was gone. Insofar as I was able to, I had shared with this girl everything that mattered to me, what the blockages were, how I was going to deal with them and what a life with me might look like. I wanted to share all of my weakness, all of my failures, all of my fears and all the good bits too. However, I continued to work ridiculous hours and to her I seemed just to be adding to that with my work on television.

I had tried to explain to her why I was doing all of this. I wanted to make the world a better place for animals and for medicine, to give animals a fair deal, to show that the love between an animal and a human can make the world better, and to bring children into a better world where I'd made a real and tangible difference in my lifetime. I wanted that to be alongside her and I absolutely wanted the best for her too, but she couldn't wait as long as that might take. She needed someone who could be there for her more than I was, which was fair enough, though heartbreaking. A time with more time for her seemed ever further away and other doubts and fears had by then got in the way for her. Maybe I should have done or said more, but at that moment all those things just wrapped like barbed wire around my heart. I know it's a cliché but somehow I had hoped that our paths were inexorably woven, one strand nowhere near as strong without the other, but both intertwined stronger and heading in the same direction.

The ghosts and demons that I've carried with me through-out my life came to visit on that barren Welsh mountainside.

I was sorry for any pain I had ever caused and I was sad because of the pain that stayed inside me. Suddenly I was like a child again and I felt desolate and worthless. Keira licked the tears off my face and in that moment she seemed to say that she knew I wasn't perfect, that I had messed up, that I was messed up, but that it wouldn't feel this bad forever.

Thank you, Keira, for soothing my heart and teaching me about love. Unconditional love.

CHAPTER FIFTEEN

Enzo and Oscar

The Field of Dreams and The Bionic Vet

Enzo Anselmo Ferrari, Enzo for short, was carried yelping and struggling into my consulting room in September 2003. The best friend of radio presenter Chris Evans, he was a four-year-old German shepherd who had been running around like the Ferrari he was named after, but had suddenly collapsed, his back legs becoming progressively paralysed. Fitzpatrick Referrals was still, at that time, operating inside Hunters Lodge primary care practice, in a residential street in Guildford. I examined him and carried out a myelography study in which we took some X-ray pictures with dye injected around his spinal cord. It became clear that he had exploded a disc in the middle of his spine – the pulpy centre of the disc had leaked out, called an acute extrusion – which compressed his spinal cord. I operated immediately.

I met Chris for the first time a few days later. I found his exuberant personality, enthusiasm for living, disarming smile, incisive intelligence and quick wit captivating and infectious. Nobody, including myself, could have guessed, from that first meeting, what a positive impact this lovely man and his family would have on my life. Nor could either of us have anticipated that the journey for Enzo would be so torturous. This would not only cement a growing friendship between Chris and I, but also chart a course that would culminate in my television career.

Enzo made a full recovery from his first surgery, but sadly, in 2008, two weeks after Fitzpatrick Referrals had moved from our interim home in Tilford to our new facility in Eashing, Enzo was rushed back into my consulting room. He was unable to stand, was dragging his back legs and could barely feel his back toes. I knew it was looking bad, but I didn't know just how bad. Fortunately, we could perform a high-powered MRI scan immediately, since myelography was by then obsolete – in any case it would have been nowhere near as sensitive in detecting his pathology. Four-and-a-half years had passed since I'd first operated on Enzo and, unfortunately, he now had three separate but related problems in the middle of his spine. First, he had suffered a huge disc explosion (extrusion) where a chronically bulging disc (protrusion) had finally ruptured and released its pulpy centre up and against his spinal cord, badly squashing it. Then, in front of this, was chronic scar tissue from the previous disc extrusion and, finally, behind this was a huge chronic protruded disc, which was also compressing his spinal cord. This kind of spinal cord injury is called 'acute-on-chronic', meaning that the disc bulge had been happening for a long time for genetic reasons and the explosion had happened suddenly. On top of Enzo's previous adjacent injury, this did not bode well.

In acute-on-chronic injuries, often a dog can cope reasonably well for some time, with just some stiffness or a reluctance to jump, for example. Then an acute extrusion of the disc on top of the chronic protrusion can damage the cord to such an extent that it may not recover. Poor Enzo had the perfect bad storm: in spite of two surgeries to remove the disc material compressing his spinal cord and to fuse solid that segment of his spinal vertebrae, his cord had been very badly compromised, and his prognosis was very unpredictable.

The spinal cord is a unique organ consisting of many hundreds of thousands of individual nerve cells, all lined up side by side, with their top ends in the brain and their tail ends reaching sometimes as far down as the lower back – which could be about 50 centimetres in a dog like Enzo. Imagine that the brain is like an electrical plug, with wires coming out of it, encased in different-coloured plastics, and these individual wires are, in turn, surrounded by a black plastic tube. The coloured plastic around each nerve is called myelin and the black plastic tube around the spinal cord is called the meninges. Just as with both the wire and the plastic in an electrical cable, if the nerves and the myelin in the spinal cord are damaged, because they are all lined up side by side, the spinal cord can't easily heal by recruiting function from neighbouring cells – unlike the cells of the liver might be able to do, for example. We are only born with one set of nerve cells with very limited capacity to regenerate if injured. With severe damage, spinal cord nerves may never recover at all, and then, as with the location and severity of Enzo's injury, the back legs which they power may never work again.

For five months, Enzo came a few times each week to our physiotherapy and hydrotherapy centre. He kept fighting with all the determination of a Formula One champion, and Chris was brave, patient, tenacious and totally dedicated to his friend's rehabilitation. We were all willing and praying for biology to smile and for Enzo's back legs to motor once more.

Then, one day, Enzo got distressed in the hydrotherapy pool and it was immediately apparent that he had twisted his stomach and spleen (gastric dilatation-volvulus), which isn't uncommon in large-breed, deep-chested dogs. I operated immediately to remove his spleen, twist his stomach back into position and stitch it down into place. Enzo, who was always such an upbeat fellow, bounced back yet again from this setback. We continued his rehabilitation as fervently as we could and he was a real trouper. Sadly, though, in the end, he never regained the use of one of his back legs. Chris even provided him with wheels to support his back end, on which he happily ran with the number plate 'Enzo' proudly displayed at his tail.

In spite of Chris and the whole team working really hard with Enzo's physio and hydrotherapy, his spinal cord injury was just too severe and he never sufficiently recovered to provide him with a great quality of life. In the end, we all had to accept that we had done our very best, and collectively we reached the decision that we had come to the end of the track. It was gut-wrenchingly sad. Chris held Enzo in his arms, I gave him an injection and we allowed him to pass away – a more kind, considerate, loving daddy he could not have had. We all miss him and he remains in our hearts forever.

No matter how many times I have had to go through such loss in my career, it still affects me deeply – in this case, all the more so, because I had got to know and respect Chris so much. A surgeon called René Leriche once said; 'Every surgeon carries about him a little cemetery, in which from time to time he goes to pray, a cemetery of bitterness and regret, where he seeks the reason for certain of his failures.' I visit those tombstones regularly in my head and each weighs like a stone on my heart.

I knew when I was building my new facility at Eashing that it would bring happiness and sadness in equal measure, that I would endure defeat, as well as rejoice in success, and that all of it was fleeting. I would never be attached to the bricks and mortar, but rather to the revolution of love and medicine that I hoped we would build inside. I love the 1989 movie *Field of Dreams* and I have always believed that if I built it, then the right thing will happen, and to paraphrase the voice speaking to Kevin Costner in the film, 'they will come'. I firmly believe that if you put enough good light out there, then others who resonate with you will come, and somehow, against all of the odds, the light gets stronger. Thus, in building the best facility that I could afford, it was my hope that the greater good might prevail and that we would be able to save as many animals and provide hope and peace for as many families as possible.

Fitzpatrick Referrals' new orthopaedic and neurosurgical centre in Eashing, my field of dreams where *The Supervet* is today filmed, opened its doors for the very first time on 24 March 2008, the day after the earliest Easter Sunday in nearly one hundred years. A few months later, the Duke of Kent formally opened the hospital. His words were most kind and encouraging, but at the time of moving in, the buildings weren't finished because of endless construction and planning issues. It took more than two years to get enough elements of the planning permission sorted for us to provide adequate parking facilities for both staff and patients' families, and also to get the go-ahead to partially power the premises with solar panels. I'm incredibly grateful to the local councils of Guildford and Waverley for allowing me to build my dream, for without their help, Fitzpatrick Referrals would not exist.

Together with my team of twenty-seven, we worked harder than ever before in our hut in the woods to fund the rest of the build and fit it out. Initially, the bank loaned me enough to rebuild only two of the four abandoned farm buildings on the site; then construction ground to a halt because I ran out of money. This was a very stressful time and there were moments when I wondered if I'd have the strength to carry on. Thankfully, however, we turned a corner, and the revenue stream generated at Tilford secured another loan with a new bank to obtain the freehold, finish the first two buildings and fund the conversion of the third building of the derelict farm. This was lucky because the third building was a dilapidated, dirty, asbestos-covered barn at the entrance of the site, which, needless to say, did not make the best first impression for potential clients.

At the time of opening, this third building wasn't finished, but it looked acceptable from the outside, so we moved in. I was adamant that there would never be bars on cages in the kennel wards and that they must be constructed of bacteria-resistant, clean-down surfaces and hardened glass doors. I also insisted on a specifically designed air-conditioning system to try to minimise the spread of bacteria, and the installation of radio and television units for the animals. In this way, I hoped to somewhat replicate some of my patients' home environments while maintaining a high level of hygiene. I wanted to make it as much of a home-away-from-home as possible. The bank wasn't happy with the extra expenditure, but I felt with certainty that the dogs and cats would be. Even today I marvel at how much less barking there seems to be when ambient daylight and calming sounds flow through the wards and I am convinced that the absence of cage bars makes a great difference to the psychological well-being of the animals in our care. I am also of the view that healing of the 'soul' is important alongside the surgical intervention that we perform. I often say that 'hugs are half of healing', in whatever form they take. I know that's true when I have had anything wrong with me.

However, the scientifically quantifiable part of healing at our new facility would take more than hugs and would depend on the best state-of-the-art equipment I could afford, and the greatest team that I could assemble. The most exciting moment of the entire build was the arrival of the MRI (magnetic resonance imaging) scanner from Germany, in which Enzo was scanned. This went into a very special room lined with a wire mesh (Faraday cage) to prevent interference from any radio frequencies outside the room, such as from television or aircraft, for example. Make no mistake, not all MRI or CT scanners are the same: you get what you pay for. After spending my summer in America all those years ago as a student working on an MRI atlas, having studied for a qualification in imaging, and having worked with various types of scanners through the years, I knew my apples from my oranges, so to speak: both round – but entirely different fruits! I also built a room big enough to house the best CT scanner I knew I'd be able to buy in the future – I couldn't afford to purchase it at the time.

For Enzo and for many animals we scan on a daily basis, an MRI scan tells us a vast amount of information about body organs. In Enzo's case, it was the degree of compression of the spinal cord, what was compressing it and what the cord itself looked like, all of which helped us to make far more accurate judgements than we were able to when I'd first treated Enzo and had only myelography as the diagnostic tool.

An MRI scanner is a giant cylindrical superconducting electromagnet. When the patient is put into the centre of the magnet, all the hydrogen protons – effectively water molecules – in the body are aligned in the same direction. During each scanning sequence, different 'slices' of imaging can be obtained, like slicing a loaf of bread. A radio-frequency pulse is fired through a wire coil in order to disrupt these protons off the line of the magnetic field. When the radio-frequency pulse is removed, the protons go back into the alignment of the magnetic field again, but the rate at which they do varies – this variable 'decay' is unique to each tissue, and the signal can be detected and recorded by the scanner to create an intensity map. Using sophisticated software algorithms, the scanner is able to convert this map into a digital image, with each different tissue type represented by a different shade of grey on the final image. Many different input frequency cocktails are tailored to show different structures to best effect, which gives rise to different kinds of maps of the body-slice scanned. In Enzo's case, for example, we could obtain a detailed picture of the cerebrospinal fluid, white and grey matter, all important constituents of the spinal cord. In this way, a three-dimensional picture of any organ can be built, and searching for disease is like looking for a single crumb by slicing a loaf of bread into very thin slices, front to back, top to bottom and side to side.

CT (computed tomography) scanners are entirely different because the image is comprised of many X-ray pictures taken at a rapid rate and reconstructed in three dimensions. The X-ray machine and the X-ray detectors for the image produced are mounted opposite each other on a circular gantry, like a doughnut, and the machine spins very rapidly around the patient. The X-rays are focused in a beam through the body as it slides through the doughnut gantry and are collected by the detectors at the end of their path. Our current scanner is capable of producing 160 images for each single rotation of the X-ray machine and produces scans at a much quicker rate than the initial six-slice scanner that we started out with. On our larger patients, scans can sometimes consist of 2–3,000 X-ray images. Advanced software reconstructs these images in three dimensions, determining the location of different body structures, which are displayed as greyscale images. X-rays travelling through more dense structures, like bone, will have their path blocked to a greater extent, resulting in only a small amount reaching the detector and thereby showing up whiter; whereas X-rays travelling through less dense structures, like lung, will mostly be allowed to pass through, showing as more black on the image. Unlike with MRI scans, CT scans, even with myelographic X-ray dye, cannot see within the spinal cord itself.

Technological advances in CT have also allowed us to increase resolution and reduce both artefact and X-ray dosage, to give us far more detailed images. Metal artefact reduction has changed my life because it allows me to look at how bone grows into metal, which until recently wasn't possible. Artefact, in this context, is the effect on the image of the scatter of the X-ray beam by the dense metal which results in 'drop out' that gives a kind of black halo around the implant, precluding visibility of the bone-implant inter-face. This certainly wasn't available back in 2008 when I saw Enzo, but in his case sadly would not have altered the out-come anyway, since his irreparable damage was within the structure of the spinal cord itself. When metal is present, we don't use MRI scans to look at the spinal cord in the region of the metal because the magnetic field is too distorted by the implants to give a clear enough image. In addition, the metal can warm up, or even move, due to the extremely powerful magnetic field. Whereas we could scan the entire spine of a German shepherd dog using our newest CT scanner in less than twenty seconds, for MRI, each individual body part must be specified in the scanner and sequences can take much longer to acquire, sometimes over an hour, even with a high-strength magnetic field.

There's a perception that all scans obtained from all scanners are the same, but that's not true. I always recommend that people check the power of the scanner and the value-for-money of the information they're paying for with their vet. This is important. Apart from the fact that very few people understand whether they should have an MRI or a CT scan for themselves, let alone their animal friend, I see families paying the same amount for scans irrespective of the power of the machine or the skill and experience of the technician manning it. A less powerful machine will provide significantly less diagnostic information by comparison with a high-powered scanner. I think everyone should ask questions. For example, is a scan, in fact, necessary at all or would a plain X-ray picture (radiograph) suffice? And, if a scan is needed, what type should be taken and why? Is it going to be low- or high-resolution? Is a qualified radiographer going to perform the scan and a qualified radiologist interpret it? And is the billing fair and proportionate to that particular quality of scan, on that particular scanner, and for an accurate interpretation of it?

A scan report is only as good as the clinical exam and the consequent medical or surgical decisions that go alongside it – in other words, a holistic view of the patient must be taken.

I constantly advise my interns and residents not to operate on the basis of a scan, but rather as indicated by patient need. For example, many dogs and humans have dried-out discs that bulge, including myself, in fact, but certainly not all cases need surgery. I can only hope that's the case for myself.

In order to make decisions appropriate for their circumstances, I think that clients should be informed of the cost of imaging relative to the cost of potential treatment. Of course, I recognise that these decisions are subjective and undoubtedly everyone involved in such a situation is doing their best, even if I feel compelled to at least illuminate the issue. The flipside is that sometimes MRI scans for example can prompt a judgment not to operate because the situation is so bleak and a decision may be made for euthanasia. As another example, with regard to CT scans, the type of surgery I perform on dogs affected by developmental elbow disease has changed vastly with advances in image quality, and this has definitely contributed to alleviating pain by providing solutions hitherto unavailable. Simply stated, I believe that we have a moral obligation to be transparent at all times and also that the families of animals should be offered the option to have potential surgery performed under the same anaesthetic as imaging, so as to save costs and time. I have seen both cancer and spinal injury patients undergo imaging, only for there then to be a significant delay before surgical intervention, which can mean the difference between therapeutic success and failure.

Although in the end we had to say goodbye to Enzo, Chris accepted that there is no guaranteed outcome with medical or surgical intervention. In my heart and in my documented medical notes, I am personally and professionally confident that I have always done my very best, and acted with the very best of intentions, but biology is a difficult master who sometimes doesn't smile. Following unsuccessful outcomes, the psychological distress for myself and my team is considerable. We have a moral and legal duty to comfort and attend to the needs of understandably distressed families, to support them through their grief and to help them find peace and acceptance that all of us have done our best but it just wasn't to be. This area of mental health for both veterinary professionals and for the guardians of animals is under-appreciated, I feel. I have certainly seen that grief can lead to a prolonged period of support, dialogue and seeking for answers, answers that are usually attributable to the vagaries of biology and unfortunate circumstance. However, I think it's true to say that these very challenging times can actually take me and my team away from treating other animals. I feel this warrants consideration in the context of the perception of failure, blame and collective moral responsibility when fully informed volitional consent – including explanation of all other available options – has led to the choice of a surgical procedure by the guardian of an animal, which sadly did not result in the outcome that anyone would have wanted. The truth is that there is no surgery that can be performed in human or animal patients without risk. In veterinary surgery, I feel that this risk should be appreciated and respected by the families of the animal consenting to the surgery in the first place, just like vets adhere to our own professional ethics, in explaining all of the options and the intended intervention. In my view, we are all on this journey together, we should all support each other, and we should always do the right thing by the patient – and by each other.

I absolutely believe in looking in the mirror following suboptimal outcomes of any intervention, but when things do not go according to plan, I can honestly say that having my heart broken by the emotions of a family who channel their grief towards me and my team is among the most difficult challenges of my life. Since being in the public eye, this criticism has intensified and found a bigger voice. I just wish that sometimes, instead of channelling their negativity towards us, people could just admit: 'I'm in extreme pain. I know that you care. Please help me to cope with my grief,' and I would move heaven and earth to do so.

Chris has given me some marvellous advice down the years, regarding this and the other challenges that sometimes overwhelm me. He has tried to teach me not to wire myself into the negativity of others, and that when I connect to what really matters to me, the right things will come my way. He has encouraged me to always try to see it from the point of view of whoever else is involved, to always do the right thing, to be at peace with myself and to realise that both criticism and praise are transient. He has taught me not to dwell on things outside of my control, or on the past, and that all things are sent to us for a reason that will ultimately be good for us. He has also encouraged me to learn from nature, and imparted one of his favourite quotes of inspiration to me: 'the sun never asks the earth for thanks'. He reminds me to do everything with good intent and never to seek out acknowledgement, praise or thanks – something our mothers taught us independently. Chris never asks for thanks, but I want to thank him anyway – and acknowledge that my life would be immeasurably poorer without his friendship.

While Enzo was swimming in the hydrotherapy pool, during his rehabilitation in 2008, Chris and I used to sit and talk in the little kitchen next to my office, and it was there that I first discussed with him the idea of making a TV programme. I wanted to tell stories about hope and redemption through the eyes of every animal that came into my vet practice, and also through the hearts of every person who loved them. I saw, over and over, the incredibly important bond of unconditional love between a human and an animal, and witnessed how, in times of crisis, whether it be illness or injury, this bond intensified. I wanted to show real-life journeys of families and their animals, to show compassion in a new way and to reflect advances in medical and surgical practice through that prism. My aim was to tell a story about love and medical science side by side. I wanted to channel positivity and goodness to show how we could achieve a better world for man and animal alike.

The series title, *The Bionic Vet*, became clear to us both during our kitchen talks, where I told Chris about the operations that I had first begun to perform in Tilford to save the legs of dogs and cats using bionic implants. These surgeries, which I continued in Eashing, by then included an array of customised options for the treatment of spinal and joint diseases, trauma and for saving limbs.

Chris took the pitch for the series to Jay Hunt, at the BBC, and discussions began that would lead to the commissioning of a series of six programmes. I had already filmed some relevant footage with Jim Incledon, whom I had met through *Wildlife SOS*, a wonderful cameraman and visionary director, passionate about the welfare of animals. These early tasters would serve as the basis for a programme idea built alongside the production company Wild Productions and its director Simon Cowell (no, not *the* Simon Cowell!). It took several months to hire a crew and get wheels set in motion. The series eventually aired on BBC 1.

Unlike *The Supervet*, which is a combination of fixed-rig

cameras and roving cameramen, *The Bionic Vet* was filmed by just three cameramen who lived on site morning, noon and night. Initially, it took some getting used to, but gradually the crew became part of the fabric of the Fitz-family practice and we all got on very well, developing great trust and respect and a real sense of camaraderie on this journey into uncharted waters. We wanted to make a veterinary programme that was quite different to anything that had gone before, where both success and failure were shown as part of everyday life, within the context of advancing medical and surgical endeavour and striving to do the right thing for the animals we love.

Many clients were asked if they would like to take part, and some said yes. I am hugely grateful to all of them for sharing their journeys. I firmly believed then, with *The Bionic Vet*, as I do now, with *The Supervet*, that the legacy of each of these stories far transcends anything I have been able to achieve by trying to advance science alone. I have authored or co-authored more than seventy academic papers on advances in veterinary medicine and delivered hundreds of academic lectures globally. It's important to emphasise that it is very necessary to provide peer-reviewed evidence for any new technique, but when *The Bionic Vet* was first broadcast on 30 June 2010, I could share for the first time with the wider world both the transformative power of the human–animal bond and how medical science might move forward, to the mutual benefit of all animals and all humans.

Jim Incledon happened to be filming at the practice when a very unlucky black cat called Oscar was referred to me for treatment in October 2009. Oscar's story would ultimately be told in episode one. A beautiful, cuddly, black domestic short-hair, not quite two years of age, Oscar was flown in from Jersey as an emergency. He had crossed the path of a combine harvester in a field, which had cut off both of his back feet below the ankles. He was desperately trying to walk on his stumps but they were sore and painful. Human amputees can often cope well on stump socket prostheses – silicone-lined sockets fitted to the stump, to which a limb is attached – and some even run, as we have seen at the Paralympics and Invictus Games. However, some struggle to cope due to pressure sores on their stumps, like my poor Uncle Paul in my childhood. Discomfort from these sores can limit mobility, and for many years the Holy Grail has been to achieve direct skeletal fixation with a metal device (endoprosthesis) that could reliably be implanted into the bone, with skin growing over it as a permanent seal against bacteria, and onto which an artificial limb (exoprosthesis) can be attached. Together the endo- and exoprostheses constitute a bionic limb. This had been my aim for our animal friends ever since I went fishing with Uncle Paul and knocked his wooden leg overboard all those years ago.

It would have been very difficult for Oscar to cope with stump socket prostheses, not to mention challenging to keep them from falling off both back legs, and by the time he was referred, I had already partnered with Professor Gordon Blunn and his associates to operate using endo- and exoprostheses on two dogs, Storm and Coal, in my previous premises.

I fused Oscar's two main ankle bones together – the talus and the calcaneus – and implanted titanium alloy pegs with porous flanges onto which the bone and the skin could grow. We then attached some small stumpy feet made with rubber and the corks from wine bottles and, by the following day, Oscar was up and about, attempting to run. Of course, it took several weeks for the bone and skin to heal, but the procedure was a success, and when he went home, his exo-prostheses were lovely white blades with black soles. He was soon back creating mayhem again, pain-free and with eight lives still intact.

Oscar was the first patient in the world, human or animal, to have two simultaneous bionic endoprostheses fitted, and that heralded a new era of possibility. Oscar went on to walk and run more or less normally with full ankle function until seven years later, when sadly one of his implants failed. We could have cut off his ankle and placed a new implant further up in his tibia, but he was managing well on one back leg and has continued to do so until this day.

As in the case of Enzo and Chris, Oscar's family realised that we were doing our very best with the techniques and im-plants of the time and, when one implant ultimately did not survive, we stood side by side, knowing we had collectively done everything we could. There are few medical successes that do not stand on the shoulders of failure. To progress, both the public and the profession must accept this unpalat-able truth, or otherwise we stand still and accept the status quo, without any advancement, which surely is unconscion-able. The corollary, of course, is that no progress can ever be made unless one patient's family consents to be the first. In most cases, innovation is born of frustration and lack of availability of other good options to provide quality of life. Some will feel that amputation prostheses or other advances for animal surgery, some of which I have introduced, are a step too far, but I believe that time will prove differently. The legacy of both Enzo and Oscar is that they have inspired future generations of implants that may help other animals and humans, as they themselves were helped.

The failure of Oscar's implant, as well as many other

successes and failures since then, has gone on to inform the design of a new invention called a PerFiTS (Percutaneous Fixation To the Skeleton), which we hope will represent a real step forward, both figuratively and literally, for animal and human amputees.

This has been a team effort by Professor Gordon Blunn, myself and a wonderful and talented engineer called Jay Meswania who is integral to the efforts of the company Fitz-Bionics, which I set up to make custom implants for animals in need. I have my dear friend and collaborator Dr Matthew Allen to thank for the rather serendipitous name of this implant, which he and I came up with one evening while he was faculty at The Ohio State University. He has since helped me considerably to advance the concepts of One Medicine, and is a scientific genius and a man of immense integrity who has been a really important companion on an often difficult journey. He continues to contribute to the future of veterinary and human medicine and is now based at The University of Cambridge veterinary school.

Through our successes and failures, we have learned that there are many factors that need to be taken into consideration, depending on the anatomical location of the implant and the species into which it is placed. By accumulating all of this information with regard to the location, type and thickness of bone and skin – for example, the shin bone of a Great Dane is very different to the ankle of a cat – we have evolved better endoprostheses over time. This knowledge will not only help other animals, but humans too. If we develop a new technique to operate on an animal that has very limited other options, all of which are suboptimal, and the family of that animal has made the considered choice to have that operation performed, the legal framework in the UK is that we may then proceed, because even if this animal is case number one, it is 'an act of clinical veterinary practice', under the Veterinary Surgeons Act, as long as all other options and potential risks have been clearly explained. The legal position is that the guardian of the animal must be presented with all of the facts as we know them at that point in time, and give *fully informed volitional consent*.

In so doing, we may help that animal, and also learn to help other animals – and humans too. Why, then, would we induce that same disease in an otherwise healthy experimental animal to learn what we already know, or repeat the mistakes of the past in either veterinary or human medicine by not learning from this new experience? The experimental animal route has until recently been the only mechanism for the development of most of the drugs and implants that humans use. I believe that we are at a crossroads, where we now have the ability to make a choice to work together – or to stay walking our separate paths in veterinary and human medicine. I see no rational, ethically well-founded reason to always choose an experimental animal model, who is then sacrificed for our benefit, over an animal transparently treated with integrity as an act of fully informed clinical veterinary practice, to save an animal who may otherwise suffer or be put to sleep.

Sadly, although both *The Bionic Vet*, and subsequently *The Supervet,* have demonstrated many examples of success and failure with limb amputation prostheses, popularly called 'bionic limbs', very little of what I have shown on television has yet filtered through into more widespread use, either in veterinary or human patients. In the former, full limb amputation is still the norm, in spite of stump socket prostheses being recommended for some patients, as far back as 1906 in

Frederick T. G. Hobday's *Surgical Diseases of the Dog and Cat*. In human medicine, meanwhile, the conventional paradigm is that experimental animal models inform progress in clinical patients, rather than the technology being deployed for animals needing treatment for their ailments. In 2010, I published the results of my initial operations on Storm, Coal and other dogs in a well-respected veterinary journal, using the implant adapted from Gordon Blunn's work, but I suspect that that paper hasn't been read by many human orthopaedic surgeons; most probably, they don't even know it exists.

It remains a great sadness for me that veterinary and human medicine haven't benefited equally from each other down the years. Though programmes like *The Bionic Vet* and *The Supervet* have, I believe, done more to raise awareness and change public perceptions than anything I can do academically. However, I have yet to inspire real and tangible change in the practical application of these techniques in animals or humans. In the veterinary world, most dogs and cats indeed function very well and have an excellent quality of life on three legs, but some don't, and they would find it even more difficult on two legs; while in the world of human medicine, using experimental animal models – rather than treating clinical animals actually affected by the disease – has been the accepted norm for more than a hundred years. However, fuelled by public awareness and collective compassionate conscience, I hope that the tide may be about to turn.

I have tried to channel my frustration regarding lack of cooperation between animal and human medicine into proactive work towards a more joined-up approach in several research fields, including spinal problems and amputation prostheses, similar to those needed by Enzo and Oscar, respectively. At The Ohio State University Spine Research Institute, in Columbus, in conjunction with Dr William Marras and his team, I am enrolled in a long-term study in which my own spine is being mapped, using MRI and CT scans over several years, alongside data on how I move while I perform surgery. This is known as kinematics: reflective balls are put on my body and motion-capture cameras follow my movement in three dimensions. (A similar technique is used in CGI in movies; for example, when the actor Andy Serkis is transformed into Gollum in *The Lord of the Rings*.) By combining this data with basic science, such as finite element modelling of vertebrae bones, along with an understanding of muscle geometry, forces and electrical activity (electromyography), the goal is to build my spine, and others, inside a computer.

I sponsored a project to lay the basic foundation to do the same for dogs. In this way, the hope is that a computer model can show age-related degeneration over time, and then we can potentially operate on this model inside the computer (in silico), and possibly create a 'surgical time machine' – which would act like a simulator enabling us to fast-forward and reverse disease processes, depending on what intervention we perform inside the computer-generated model. Nobody nowadays would buy a new car that hadn't been crash-dummy tested; yet we have surgery that hasn't been rehearsed inside a computer. In the future, I hope we can model the kind of disease Enzo had, and I also have in my discs and vertebrae, in tandem on a computer. I hope we can learn from each species so that we can be more accurate in our choice of surgical intervention. That is why I myself am part of the experiment that may ultimately help animals and humans, too. How otherwise will we ever know which treatment may be best for a given set of circumstances, except by sacrificing more experimental animals? Computer-modelling and other emerging research technologies can, I hope, over time significantly reduce reliance on experimental models.

I realised long ago that I would make little difference in my life unless I could understand and communicate through the heart rather than through the mind alone. An understanding of rational science rarely changes the world just on its own, unless people respond and connect on an emotional level. *A picture paints a thousand words*, they say – and so it was with Oscar, whose impact was huge for the general public. This little black cat with his white blade feet appeared first on *The Bionic Vet*, before capturing public hearts and imagination through his picture in newspapers across the globe, from the *Himalayan Times* to the *Irish Times*, and almost every publication in between. He shone a light on science that the public would never otherwise have been aware of. Suddenly, it seemed *The Bionic Vet* was on the map and it became popular in many countries around the world.

The Bionic Vet and the doors it has since opened, including a growing awareness of the value of veterinary and human medicine working together, in a cohesive platform of One Medicine, would not have occurred without Enzo and Chris Evans coming into my life – and without a revolution in biological engineering that, in turn, had been made possible by the combination of advanced imaging and engineering. For the first time in veterinary medical history, we can manufacture three-dimensional implants using CT scans and interrogate the body in minute detail using MRI scans. It has become possible with metal artefact reduction on CT scans to track how bone grows into implants, potentially obviating the need to sacrifice an experimental animal in order to prove that implants work. All of this has happened within a decade. In 2009, at the time of filming *The Bionic Vet*, I founded FitzBionics with Jay Meswania, and since then we have created dozens of bionic solutions where they hadn't existed before.

A new era was dawning and, in 2010, it felt like the effort of building my field of dreams was going to be worth it. The following years would prove challenging and frustrating, though, as I set out to forge a new future for both education and medicine by trying to build two more hospitals, study for further exams to become a recognised specialist and help to found a new veterinary school in the UK, alongside a charitable foundation to further the principles of One Medicine.

Enzo and Oscar were catalysts for positive change. Enzo brought Chris and me together and, for the rest of my life, I shall remain grateful to that wilful, joyous, brave fluff-ball of wagging tail and gnawing teeth. Enzo's legacy is that Chris and I became and remain the best of friends. Oscar opened a portal in public perception and awareness that can never be closed again – if a cat can run on skeleton-anchored bionic legs, then so can a man or woman.

Thank you, Enzo and Oscar, for shining a radiant light into my life, which illuminates the path ahead.

CHAPTER SIXTEEN

Tiger

Life, Death, Exams and Other Stresses

After the temporary media whirlwind of *The Bionic Vet* in 2010, I knuckled down to try to make our new adventure in Eashing as successful as it could possibly be. I had two primary aims for Fitzpatrick Referrals: to become a certified boarded specialist surgeon myself so I could best lead my growing team, and to extend our hospitals from one to three centres so that we could encompass the surgical disciplines of cancer, soft-tissue surgery and regenerative medicine, in addition to orthopaedics and neurosurgery.

It felt like I was falling at the first hurdle in May 2013, when two months before my specialist examinations, I was dying of stress, trying to juggle practice commitments and find time to study. Then one day, everything was drawn into sharp perspective. My dedicated and dependable surgical resident, Padraig, had driven to Devon to collect an emergency case, a cat called Tiger. His family thought that he had been caught in some kind of trap or snare because there were noose marks around the bottoms of both back legs and his tail. The bottom of his left back leg was gangrenous, the bottom of his right back leg was very swollen and, because the blood supply had been cut off, most of his tail was dead. Initially, we considered a limb amputation prosthesis surgery for his left back leg, but then the right back leg improved and we intended to proceed with the amputation of his left back leg and his tail instead – the likelihood was that he would be perfectly happy on three legs, as many cats are.

Unfortunately, Tiger's heart suddenly stopped after an anaesthetic, when he was recovering in the wards. This can happen to any animal, or human, but thankfully it is a very rare event. He was rushed to the emergency area and the team began resuscitation with chest compressions, desperately trying to get his heart beating again. This didn't work, and by the time the team had called me, and I ran down from my office upstairs, minutes had passed and adrenaline had been administered, but there was still no response. The seconds were ticking by and he had flatlined on the electrocardiogram. Drugs and thoracic compressions were not working – and time was running out.

It is always very difficult to make the decision to perform open cardiac compressions, especially as even this had not been successful for a previous patient, in spite of my best efforts. But with Tiger, my judgement was that we'd tried chest compressions for long enough and he wasn't responding – so I made the call. In a matter of seconds, we clipped the side of the chest, sterilised as best we could, and I grabbed a scalpel blade and cut. I opened Tiger's chest between the ribs over the heart, just enough to get my index finger in, and I started to pump. The count commenced, all eyes on the monitor. The aim in such an extreme circumstance is to apply about 110 compressions per minute to the heart. One. Two. Three. Four. Five. Six—.

The next two minutes seemed like an eternity. Several nurses and interns huddled around doing whatever they could – or just hoping and praying. A feeling of foreboding hung on the air as we all counted and I pumped his little heart. I kept asking for a pulse: still nothing. Again: nothing. The nurse shook her head sadly to my increasingly urgent, repeated question. I was on the point of admitting defeat and thought that we'd lost him, but then a miracle. I thought I could feel Tiger's heart beat once on its own. I hardly dared to hope, and then it happened again and yet again – three times, then I was sure. It was as if I could actually feel the electricity flowing back into the heart, pulse by pulse. We held our breath in suspended animation, hardly believing what we were witnessing, but it was true: Tiger was back! He had cheated death.

We stitched up his chest then everyone looked at the ECG monitor in anxious silence. Tiger really had come back to life and we at last exhaled, as if we'd been holding our breath for hours. If Tiger's heart had stopped for any longer, he would almost certainly be either permanently brain-damaged or dead. As it was, that didn't happen and, after we amputated Tiger's leg and tail, he made a full recovery and returned to his erstwhile crazy ways, climbing roofs and trees. That moment, when Tiger's heart started beating again, was profound for all of us. At times like that one, the tenuous hold that we all have on life is brought home in a big way. It's seldom that one gets reminded in such a dramatic fashion that life and death are literally in one's hands as a veterinary surgeon. I know for sure that whenever I do face life-or-death situations, I'm reminded how quickly life is passing for all of us and not to be attached to money, ego, power or glory because it could all be gone tomorrow.

I was emotionally and mentally going through what felt like my own 'near death' experience shortly thereafter due to the impending examinations. During the two years leading up to my specialist exams in 2013, I knew the journey would be difficult, but I had no idea just how difficult. I had the dual goal of becoming a registered specialist in veterinary orthopaedics and also a professor. Along the way, I added a third – to sit exams in America for the College of Veterinary Sports Medicine and Rehabilitation. I figured if I was studying anyway, I might as well try to make it count as much as possible.

Anyone who has ever studied for specialist examinations will tell you that it consumes your life for a couple of years, taking over a part of your brain every waking moment – and some while you're sleeping, too: it's a ticking time bomb waiting to explode, either in elation or deflation. Many people take off a few months before important exams to study, but because I was the major revenue generator in my practice, I continued to consult and operate until less than three weeks before the exams, needing to prove to the bank that their funding of the new buildings at Eashing and the proposed new hospital in Guildford were good business decisions and that they would see a return on their investment. I hoped they would then perhaps be more amenable to extending further financial backing for future projects. I'm very grateful to my interns at the time, who not only read scientific papers to me while I operated, but also congregated regularly in the lecture theatre to discuss books and papers with me, contributing to their learning and exams, as well as my own. I often thought of my daddy imparting knowledge to me in the old hay barn at home, which was similar to the one from which the lecture theatre building had been constructed. I gained comfort from the memory of his smile and his wise words that 'knowledge is no load to carry', though I often observed that it sure was challenging to store it in the brain in the first place – and it didn't get easier with age! For the final couple of weeks I was holed up in a tiny room, with diagrams and charts stuck all over the walls and the ceiling (so that I could look at them when I was lying in bed). It was as if I was reliving my student days in my Dublin bedsit.

I had put my personal life on hold for quite a while and I'm very sad that I didn't or couldn't balance commitments better, but I was consumed by what I'd committed to do. Some very special people in my life were hurt by my lack of availability for them at this time. I'm sorry if I caused them pain.

Fear and anxiety about 'brain freeze' sapped my energy day by day as the exams quickly approached. Although I had written huge folders of notes, I was convinced that I couldn't remember any of them. I made a wonderful friend at this time in Bill Oxley, who was the only other person in the UK sitting the Royal College examination that year, and was therefore the only person on earth who understood, as he was experiencing similar fears. He and I would compare notes and examine each other's knowledge, which probably scared each of us even more. This bond, forged in the purgatory of exam preparation, remains treasured by both of us, and whenever I see him again, even today, it is with a mixture of gut-churning fear and great joy that I give him a big hug. By chance, on 7 July 2013, a couple of days before my exams, I was listening to an interviewer on the news ask Andy Murray how he stayed calm before his impending Wimbledon final. He answered that he walked his dog. His answer echoed my own life – walking Keira was one of the few things to bring me solace during those final horrible days. She looked up at me from beneath her big bushy eyebrows and said in her own way: 'Don't panic, Daddy, everything will be OK in the end.' I kept trying to tell myself it actually wasn't a life or death experience, unlike poor Tiger, but while my 'sensible head' wasn't working, my 'irrational, scared' head most certainly was.

That year, Murray defeated Novak Djokovic in straight sets to win Wimbledon, but I had no such luck. I went into the Royal College of Veterinary Surgeons, where I had previously registered in 1991, with a bottomless pit in my belly. I followed the short procession of people taking various examinations into the austere, musky, wood-panelled chamber, all the while feeling the walls ominously closing in on me. Terror grabbed at every sinew in my body as I breathed deeply, sat at the desk, got my pen and pencil ready, waited for the invigulator to say 'start' and turned over the paper. I was a forty-six-year-old man with the fear of a twelve-year-old boy on his very first day in secondary school. All at once, I felt I was not good enough, brave enough, strong enough, just like that night, all those years ago, when I lost those lambs, back home in Ireland.

I looked at the questions. We had to write long essays on several topics and could only leave out one set question. There was one that I knew instantly I had to avoid – it was about a very specific paper and I just couldn't remember the details. That left me with several others that I knew I could bang out almost in a stream of consciousness. I pity the poor examiners dealing with my handwriting. Then came the crunch. I had just started a question on drawing and naming the nerves of the brachial plexus (armpit) in a dog, when it happened – brain freeze. I drew a complete mental blank, even though I could picture the very diagram on the ceiling in my bedroom and had memorised it for months. There I was, back inside my headspace in the first year of vet school when I failed the anatomy examination, because the brachial plexus just went all fuzzy in my head – and, no matter what, I simply couldn't clear the haze.

The brachial plexus comes off the spinal cord in the lower neck in any mammal and goes through a complex web of nerves to distribute down the arm like the M25 motorway around London giving off tributary roads to the south of England. I knew that neural network like the back of my hand, and had operated on it loads of times, but in that examination room, in 2013, my nerves just got the better of me and the mist became a dark, all-enveloping cloud. To make matters worse, I'd suffered from nervous diarrhoea for a couple of days before.

I asked to leave the exam room, went into the toilet and had a full-blown panic attack, the likes of which I had not experienced before – in regard to my academic life, at least. This was a whole new level of stress for me. I was sick, and afterwards sat on the toilet with my eyes closed as I banged my head against my hands. After all of the experience of and the effort involved in the previous twenty-three years to get to this point, everything hung on this one question – and I knew, but couldn't remember, the answer. I had to accept that I would probably fail the paper on the basis of not being able to access those tiny neurones in my brain which could recall SMARMU – Suprascapular, Musculocutaneous, Axillary, Radial, Median, Ulnar. I returned to my seat in the exam auditorium and scribbled something around the subject of the question in the hope of picking up a few points, but I knew that I was screwed. After the examination, I left the building in the very depths of despair and, driving home through Putney, had to pull over and run into a pub toilet to vomit my guts up, yet again.

I had to wait a few torturous weeks before sitting the second part of my examinations – the oral and practical components. My colleagues at Fitzpatrick Referrals will likely remember that month forever, as I was more depressed than I've ever been. On the drive up to Nottingham veterinary school to take my exams, all of the ghosts of my personal, academic and professional failures gnawed away at me, and I was sweating profusely and stressed beyond reason. This wasn't helped by the fact that I turned up late because I got caught in some roadworks.

I parked, shivering with trepidation, even though it was a sunny day. I opened the door of the car and a small sprig with a flower on it from a nearby tree blew down and landed at my feet, causing me to look up. There in the tree was a robin redbreast: I felt my heart suddenly lift. Then, on my walk to the examination building, I passed near a chestnut tree, another lucky sign for me. Maybe it was going to be OK after all.

A few weeks later, I was on my way to Michigan to sit my American Board Specialist examinations. I landed in East Lansing and went to get a taxi outside the airport. What must have been the rustiest cab in the state pulled up, driven by a heavily bearded guy who looked like a dude from ZZ Top. A lady, who I assumed was his wife, with a big mop of tousled hair, longer even than his beard but exactly the same colour of grey, was sitting in the passenger seat beside him, smoking a cigarette. At that very moment, a man with a massive suitcase rushed up and asked me if he could share my taxi. It turned out that he had flown in from Japan to sit the same examinations as me. Very quickly, in staccato bursts of excited speech, he told me that he was my biggest fan and had listened to all of my lectures. I was absolutely stunned and, of course, agreed to him sharing my taxi. However, there wasn't room in the back for both of our large suitcases. Mine was full of folders of notes and I suspect his was, too. I helped my new Japanese friend to position his suitcase between us on the back seat, while our driver removed an oil drum from the trunk of the car and popped my bag there instead, stashing the drum at the legs of his wife. Despite the obvious fire hazard, she lit up another cigarette. This was already not going well.

My co-passenger was hidden behind the oversized, hard plastic suitcase perched between us. He was trying to pass me his business card, all the while shouting, 'You come to Japan! You come to Japan! We love you!'

ZZ Top floored the accelerator and we careered off, his wife laughing and smoking in the front. The reason for the speedy getaway wasn't immediately apparent, until I saw the railway barrier lights ahead and an eternally long train in the distance, coming down the track to our right. Our cab zoomed across the tracks just as the barriers came down. ZZ Top jammed on the brakes, with such force that the suitcase broke through the rusty divider between the front and back of the cab, landing on the gear stick – all to great cackles of laughter from ZZ and his wife.

'Those dang trains keep passin' for half an hour, ya know. Lucky we got through,' he mumbled as he shoved the suitcase back towards us. 'Don' worry 'bout that now, boys, it was jus' waitin' to bust anyways.' This was definitely not going well.

As we stopped at the gates momentarily, I looked up and saw a poster of a man's head, with the cheesiest smile I'd ever seen – it was a dentist advertising his own services. The billboard read, 'The Number One Dentist in Michigan'. We were close enough that I could see an asterisk near this bold statement. The accompanying 'small' print at the bottom of the poster read '*according to my mum'. I kid you not. My own mammy had no tangible idea what I was doing with my life at that moment or how stressful these exams were, because I didn't like to worry her, but even if she had, she would no doubt have commented that 'pride takes a fall'. I was desperately hoping that my confidence would stay intact for these exams, and that I would pass, though I knew with certainty that I wouldn't be Number One.

I sat in my room in the Kellogg Conference Center, in East Lansing, for two days and nights before the exams, drinking instant coffee, and studying all of the folders in my bag. By the time they came around, a strange sense of calm had come over me, quite unlike my earlier experience in Nottingham. I could only do my best – what would be would be. I was nervous and yet resigned to my fate.

In the end, fate was on my side it seemed: I became a registered specialist in the UK and the US shortly there-after – somehow, I'd picked up enough marks in the clinical and practical aspects of the RCVS Diploma examinations to compensate for my mental block in the written paper. All of the sleepless nights and stressful days had been worth it, but I couldn't rest. There was too much still to do. The following day, I went straight back to work and carried on trying to achieve my other goals. From the time of my very first serious examinations in secondary school, I've never slapped myself on the back or overly rejoiced in any of my successes. I have been embarrassed to show anyone my awards or certificates, going back to that time when I hid the student of the year prize in the hay barn, all those years ago.

My specialist examinations earned 'the stripes' to prove my worth in a leadership role and I can't expect to contribute in the way I would like in my life without passing exams to prove my credentials, but I am acutely aware that the qualifying piece of paper does not make one an 'expert' or a brilliant surgeon – it just proves knowledge, not surgical acumen. Any capacity I have as a surgeon is born of an apprenticeship of purpose and is the product of experience and of caring deeply about my patients. I know many vets and nurses who don't have extra letters after their name, but do an amazing job as clinicians and surgeons with compassion and integrity. I've always seen any achievement as a stepping stone and not as a destination in itself, although I understand that each is important. While I accept that there is gratification for one's ego in getting letters after one's name, it has never been about that for me. I'm very much aware that I am passing through this world and I'm not attached to things that don't ultimately matter in the overall scheme of things.

I often rejoice more in the achievements of those I have been fortunate enough to teach and mentor than I do in my own. I guess it's a bit like having children – though I have not had that particular honour yet – in that you want your successors to take what you have learned and make an even bigger difference in the world, to carry the torch as it were. And for this reason, I set out to try to help build a new veterinary school in Surrey, where I hoped that the students would be open-minded about the concept of One Medicine and would truly seek to give animals a fair deal in every respect.

I had had the first meeting regarding this idea back in 2010, when a client, John Hay, had given me an introduction to the governing body of the University of Surrey. Through John I met with the vice-chancellor, Professor Chris Snowden, and Lisa Roberts, who was Professor of Health Sciences. Chris (now vice-chancellor of the University of Southampton) is a genius and a visionary. Finally, it seemed, I was in a room with people who understood the concept of One Medicine – that animal and human medicine could and should move forward together by learning from each other. We talked for a long time about the subject – the related potential for integration of the work that I was doing in animals with human medicine and vice versa was crystal clear to all of us.

We discussed whether a new veterinary school could be founded based on the core value that a vet's ultimate responsibility is to the animal, but how that should extend to an effort to protect the lives of every animal species globally, including the aim of reducing the need for experimental animals through a platform of One Medicine. It's extraordinary, I feel, that as vets we 'sign up' to take care of the welfare of animals but, in the main, we do so only for animals in our direct care, very rarely thinking of the welfare of wild animals or research animals sacrificed for human gain, whose sacrifice might be minimised if we opened our minds to new ways of working.

At this time, there had not been a new veterinary school since Nottingham opened in 2006, which was the first in fifty years. Student numbers in veterinary medicine in the UK were strictly controlled by central government, therefore the establishment of a new school would require the agreement of the Higher Education Funding Council for England (HEFCE), the Royal College of Veterinary Surgeons (RCVS) and the University of Surrey Council, and all of this was to prove a formidable obstacle in us going forward. In the end, it was the force of nature that is Chris Snowden, the resourceful

Lisa and John and an astute Roberto La Ragione, who joined the team and is now head of pathology at the school, who together found a way. I was on hand, whenever needed, to help push the cause a little further in the right direction, but it was these four extraordinary individuals who were responsible for founding the new vet school.

When regulations changed in 2012 and universities were no longer limited in the numbers of students they could recruit, with grades of AAB or higher, as needed in veterinary medicine, Sir Chris Snowden (he'd been knighted in the New Year's Honours for services to higher education and engineering) approached first the HEFCE, and then the RCVS, with the idea for the vet school. Once tentative support was in place, we all made presentations to the University Council. Finally, in October 2012, Surrey University announced its intention to launch the new school.

In May 2013, Chris Proudman was appointed as the first head of the Surrey School of Veterinary Medicine. I remember the buzz at the inaugural open day in 2014, when students came to see the school being built and hear of the cutting-edge practices that were to be housed within it. There were bright eyes everywhere in the audience as I took to the stage to give a lecture named in honour of one of my most important mentors, Philip Gilbert. It was called 'A Reason Big Enough' and it was as epic an occasion for me as it was for many of the young people present. I explained that the future of veterinary medicine was in their hands, as Tiger's life had once been in mine. Using examples of the various animals that I have listened to and learned from through the years, I explained how I had found my reason big enough – which on that particular day was to inspire them. Over 1,000 people applied for the new course and the original target of twenty-five students was raised to forty-five to accommodate the number of exceptionally strong candidates.

Sir Christopher wrote to the Queen in November 2014 to ask her to open the new school, recognising that her interest in education, young people and, of course, animals might perhaps secure her participation. He was right, but no doubt his charm and standing in the world of education also had a role to play in her decision.

On 15 October 2015, opening day, I rushed to the men's toilets, located behind the biggest lecture room in the new facility, knowing my nerves would inevitably make their way from my head down to my bladder. I had been there for just the briefest of moments when two suited men, wearing car wires, came in and stood one either side of me: they were the Royal Protection Squad (RPS).

'All right, Noel,' piped up one of them. I looked to my left and recognised the man, having treated one of his dogs for the Metropolitan Police. It turned out I had met both of them before – and they jokingly told me to behave myself when Her Majesty turned up. About an hour later, when I did meet the Queen, I was very well behaved indeed. I ended up explaining to her how skin and bone grew onto an amputation prosthesis device – and how this progress could help dog and man together. She was most gracious, and I felt truly honoured that she listened so intently to what I had to say about how animal and human medicine can work closer together through One Medicine. I have since been humbled to become the first professor of orthopaedics at the vet school.

Chris Snowden had a serious accident earlier in 2015, and was lucky to survive to see the Surrey School of Veterinary Medicine completed. We stood shoulder to shoulder on that day and, as the ribbon was cut, we just gave each other a nod of acknowledgement for the achievement. The gestation of the idea had come years earlier and we were both so pleased to see our dream realised and imagine the bright young minds that would find inspiration here, as the mantle of their mentorship was handed over to a wonderful leader, Chris Proudman, and his equally inspired team.

In 2010, while trying to get the new vet school off the ground, I was also trying to achieve another dream – getting the second of the three planned Fitzpatrick Referrals hospitals into existence, a specialist hub for oncology and soft-tissue surgery. This involved persuading the bank to lend me yet more money. I had already begun discussions to try to secure a piece of land on which to build my planned surgery. There was no room at the site in Eashing for a hospital of the magnitude I envisioned, so I reasoned that if I could get planning permission and cooperation from the Surrey Research Park, beside the university, then potentially we could have students accessing a state-of-the-art facility within walking distance of the veterinary school. This could expose them to world-class surgery and the philosophy of One Medicine early in their careers.

I also dreamed that one day I might be able to help the University of Surrey found a medical school so that student vets and doctors could forge lifelong friendships and professional collaborations side by side. In this way, understanding without mutual prejudice could possibly be built. On this foundation a true platform for cross-collaboration could flourish. Alas, my dream of One Medicine hasn't been realised yet, and regretfully may not be anytime soon.

Further development at Fitzpatrick Referrals was much

more within my power, though, provided that I could secure a bank loan. I wanted to gather together what I hoped would become the greatest team of clinicians in the world – a sort of veterinary *Avengers Assemble*. The practice at Eashing was growing to be part of my long-held vision for animals, inspired by Charles and William Mayo's Mayo Clinic of super-specialist hubs for humans in America. In our orthopaedics and neurology centre, clinical research and bionic regenerative technology development would fuel advance as an integral part of the plan and as in the Mayo clinic, funds would be re-invested for the greater good of the patients and clinical team.

I knew that I would need a hero of super-specialism in cancer to lead the clinical team at the second proposed hospital. There was only one man in the world who I felt could don this cape, someone whose career and academic achievements I had tracked for many years. I had seen Professor Nick Bacon lecture in the UK after he had finished his residency in small animal surgery at Cambridge, first in 2003, and then again in 2007 in Chicago, when I heard him speak about cancer. I knew instantly that he was the superhero I needed. Nick, who had gone on to work in America, had become, in my opinion, one of the greatest surgical oncologists in the world for companion animals. Finally, on 22 October 2010, at a symposium in Seattle, I was able to sit down with him in a wine bar and ask if he would like to draw his own dream oncology facility on a blank canvas. I said I would 'build it if he would come', that I believed we could change the world of vet medicine together. Soon afterwards, thankfully, he came on board. After Sarah Girling, he was my second veterinary Avenger. Now, all I needed was the money!

I was convinced that I could force the second hospital

into existence if I worked hard enough – but I was wrong. After a detailed business plan was put together, I met with representatives from my bank in the lecture theatre at the practice in Eashing, which I had built in honour of my daddy. Even though I gave the best pitch that I could, the bank officials refused, saying that they didn't think that there would be enough financial return from treating dogs with cancer or soft-tissue problems to justify another loan. I replied emphatically that I was going to make it happen with or without them. I walked down the corridor to my office and put my head in my hands. Glancing up at my daddy's dehorning saw which was framed on my wall, I remembered how he had done exactly the same when he couldn't raise the money to buy the piece of land called the Glebe. He somehow made the purchase happen so that he could nurture that land back to health and I wanted to nurture as many animals as I could back to health. I would not be defeated.

My financial controller, Dineke Abbing, watched my dejection with some trepidation; she knew I had meant what I said, and to us the plan made absolute sense. The second hospital, and in due course a third, were, in our minds, wholly necessary to create a super-specialist landscape within which all of the symbiotic disciplines of orthopaedics, neurosurgery, soft-tissue surgery, oncology and ultimately regenerative medicine could each help the other, with the goal of being among the best – if not the best – practice of our kind in the world. For my own part, I was incredulous that financiers didn't see the future of this vision with the same appetite that I had. In my head, it was completely obvious and absolutely essential. I was also quite sure that if I had not been the sole driver, and was in fact a corporate subsidiary, the money would have been found, but I wanted to be true to the vision of giving back to the animals, rather than ultimately just giving back to a financial machine. It was poor Dineke's job to help me realise this vision. Her predecessor had kept a close eye on Fitzpatrick Referrals' finances at our former practice in Tilford so that the facility at Eashing could be built, but it is Dineke who has facilitated the expansion to where we are at today, sharing all of the stress and sleepless nights with intense loyalty and tenacity. She has had to put up with more of my ups and downs than anybody else in the past decade: it is not an exaggeration to say that Fitzpatrick Referrals, as it exists today, would not have happened without Dineke at the financial helm.

All of my team have shown great resilience, determination, patience, understanding and loyalty over the years, embracing my dreams and working towards them with me. The challenges for them have been considerable, because the dream is truly massive regarding what I feel we are capable of achieving for veterinary medicine and the animal world. I do understand the material world and I'm at peace with it. I think that you deserve to have whatever you want materially as long as you're a good person, look after the folks around you and pay your dues to society. For my own part, I have, to date, only owned one material possession for pure pleasure and that was an Aston Martin Vantage. I loved that car – a sleek, black adrenaline machine on wheels. About a year after I bought it, in early 2012, I wanted to hire a resident vet, and the bank wouldn't, at the time, loan me the money to pay for the position, as they didn't see the value unless I could prove revenue generation. Of course, I couldn't. So I sold the Aston Martin and instead hired one of the best, most loyal, most hard-working, most dedicated and kindest young vets I have ever known, Susan Murphy. This young lady has proven to be worth one thousand Aston Martins, and more. I'm hugely proud of her achievements and, hopefully, she will soon be a boarded specialist surgeon.

A couple of days after my failed pitch to the bank, I got the train into the financial heart of London to present my ideas for the new hospital to venture capital groups. All the time, I could hear my daddy in my head whispering, 'never to join with anyone except in a prayer, and certainly not in business, because their motivation will never be the same as yours'. Of course, he was right.

My motivation was to treat cancer in dogs: the venture capitalists' motivation was to make money. While it was entirely understandable that financiers need to make a profit, it was, nonetheless, frustrating. I was having a very difficult time persuading anyone to take on the risk to fund my dream and the constant effort was both time-consuming and stressful, the rejections disappointing and disheartening. I just couldn't see the problem – I *knew* that if someone provided financial backing, we'd make good on it within a ten-year period, and more importantly do a lot of good along the way. No investor was prepared to take a long-term view, or consider the merits of what I was trying to do; to them it was just a business decision, which I could understand, but I couldn't relate to on any level.

Finally, Dineke and I managed to persuade a new bank to lend me enough money not just to keep the ortho-neuro practice at Eashing going, but also to build the new facility in Guildford. They didn't give me all I needed to fund a linear accelerator cyber-scalpel to cut out cancer, but I built a bunker for it anyway, just as I had done years before for the scanners at Eashing: 'build it and they will come'.

Soon afterwards, another veterinary Avenger came on

board, a very talented soft-tissue surgeon, Laurent Findji. Then Stuart Carmichael, my wonderful mentor from the early 1990s, joined us to manage the hospital build. Stuart, Nick and Laurent assembled as a formidable team to put the cancer and soft-tissue hospital on the map, and without them it would never have happened even if I had all the money in the world, because treating cancer has much more to do with the compassion and skill of the people than it will ever have to do with the building that they work in.

On 2 September 2015, Fitzpatrick Referrals Oncology and Soft Tissue Centre opened its doors. My dear friend, Chris Evans, who had encouraged me, helping to propel our work to global consciousness with *The Bionic Vet*, cut the ribbon while standing beside another man, remarkably of the same name, Professor Sir Chris Evans. A global luminary in human cancer research, Sir Chris is someone with whom I hope to travel the road towards One Medicine.

In the five years between 2010 and 2015, we laid a few of the foundation blocks on that road towards One Medicine. In addition to realising my personal ambition to specialise, we helped to found a new vet school that will hopefully inspire future generations of vets to embrace advances in animal medicine and surgery alongside those in the human medical field, and look to the welfare of all animals globally, whether directly in their care or not. As I stood in the carpark when we opened our second hospital, with my mammy and friends around me, I felt very grateful to all of the growing Fitz-family working towards better techniques and treatments, and grateful to the animals, like Tiger, who had taught me so much when I was willing to listen to them, rather than to those who said it could not be done or it wasn't worth it. Hard work, belief, faith and tenacity are worth it, and when every veterinary professional, from receptionist and ward auxiliary to veterinary nurse and veterinary surgeon, in either of our hospitals holds a paw – or a hand of someone who loves that paw – it is worth it. We see life and death every day, exams are a fleeting moment, and the other stresses are all somehow worth it in that one moment of unconditional love.

We had come a long way since I had lost the lambs in a frozen field as a child, but the vision was only beginning to take shape. To start building on these foundations, I would also need to create a platform to fund medical research that did not sacrifice animal life, through founding a charity, and I would need to capture public awareness, by getting the message of love and hope back on television.

CHAPTER SEVENTEEN

Mitzi

Becoming The Supervet through One Medicine

On a radiant sunny summer morning in June 2010, two weeks before *The Bionic Vet* was broadcast, a beautiful three-year-old white German shepherd dog called Mitzi hobbled on three legs into my consulting room. Mitzi's mum, Viv, and her daughter, Zoe, had brought her up from Dorset to see me. Mitzi had been trampled by a horse and when I sedated her and removed her bandage, it was clear that her right back foot had been almost severed and was hanging off by a sinew. Viv and Zoe were both shivering with shock and terror; they couldn't bear for her to lose the entire leg and had made the journey to the surgery in the hope that I could fit a new bionic foot into the bones of the ankle.

We had, by then, performed a number of these procedures using an endoprosthesis – an implant secured to the bone that then extends out through the skin which is stitched onto it – and an exoprosthesis foot attached to the outside. By good fortune, Mitzi's veterinary team knew about our work and referred her to see me.

Since it was effectively dead already, I amputated what remained of Mitzi's foot, obtained a CT scan of the limb, and used the three-dimensional images to design a device with Jay and Gordon, who were by now colleagues. Mitzi's personalised endoprosthesis was then implanted, just as had been done a few years earlier for Oscar the cat, by fusing the two main ankle bones (talus and calcaneus). Once the skin had healed onto the bottom of the endoprosthesis, we were able to attach a blade-shaped foot made from carbon fibre to the metal spigot sticking through the skin. Within two weeks, Mitzi could walk relatively normally and, after three months, she returned to full function. She was able to live a fully active, healthy and happy life for another six-and-a-half years.

Some people may dream of being on the cover of *Newsweek* or *Time* magazines, but when one lives in Surrey, the apogee of achievement is to be on the front page of the *Surrey Advertiser*. I was understandably very excited, therefore, when I was featured, with Mitzi the bionic dog, in a cover story. I had arrived! Or so I thought ... Since the newspaper was folded over on newsstands, with the picture of Mitzi's bionic leg on the hidden bottom half, all the reader could see on the topside was my leprechaun head beside the other headline of that week, 'Predatory Abuser Lured Girls'. It was a PR tragedy. There I was, on every newsstand in Surrey – no bionic leg, no bionic headline – just the most salacious of headlines beside what appeared to be my grinning mugshot. Ah, the cruel double-edged sword of celebrity.

My second newspaper 'experience' was altogether a more serious affair, however. I did an interview with the *Sunday Times* in which I talked in broad terms about the technology involved in Mitzi's prosthetic device, and how it potentially heralded hope and a new dawn for animal and human amputees. The same day, Professor Blunn received a phone call from the manufacturers of the implant, threatening both him and me with legal action for talking about the device, which Gordon himself had invented and which was at the time being used in human patients. The irony was, as I've mentioned before, that in February 2010 I had submitted and subsequently published a paper in the journal *Veterinary Surgery*, in which I described the very same procedure using the same technology, and illustrating exactly how the implant worked in the bone and the skin of a clinical patient.

From my perspective, it appeared that the company that was now threatening us appeared less concerned about a scientific article published in a veterinary journal than a profile in the *Sunday Times*. Perhaps they were worried that surgeons, who do not typically read the veterinary literature, might be upset if they read a *Sunday Times* article about the use of this implant in dogs, or they felt that the intellectual property associated with the implant – from which monetary gain could accrue – may be compromised, which of course wasn't the case. In lectures and in episodes of *The Bionic Vet*, Gordon and I had always been very open about our desire to collaborate and translate lessons learned from humans to dogs, and vice versa, and the newspaper article revealed no more than we had already discussed openly.

In the end, I was saddened by the attitude of the company, which to me seemed more motivated by the possibility of reputational damage or monetary gain than by doing the right thing for both human and animal patients. To add insult to injury, I had obtained informed consent from the families of these animals with full disclosure of all the risks, and I had paid the company for each of the implants used in these patients, making it very hard to argue that my use was in any way inappropriate, could bring them into disrepute, or would reveal company secrets that weren't already in the public domain. In a somewhat ironic twist of fate, we would learn from surgical challenges associated with this device and go on to develop what we hoped would be an improved implant – the PerFiTS, thus named because it came through the skin (Percutaneous) and Fixated To the Skeleton. Our goal was to constantly improve and learn from challenges that we encountered in animals and in humans, while using the device that caused this temporary kerfuffle.

The fact of the matter is that most medical advances, whether implants, prostheses, drugs or new biological therapies, need to make money for the companies that invest in their development. The costs involved in developing, testing and securing regulatory approval for new therapies can be massive, with estimates of over $1 billion for some new drugs. There is a clear need for companies to protect intellectual property and patents, because it isn't until the implant or drug is widely released that the investment in research, development, safety testing and clinical trials can start to be recouped. This is completely understandable. The tragedy is, though, that the vast majority of these drugs and implants are developed using experimental animals who have to be put to sleep at the end of the study so that companies can obtain the postmortem information needed to secure regulatory approval for the drug or device. This requirement for what is referred to as 'terminal' animal studies has been in place for many decades, and represents the best efforts of regulatory bodies – such as the Food and Drug Administration in the USA and the Medicines and Healthcare products Regulatory Agency (MHRA) in the UK – to ensure the safety of these treatments ahead of clinical trials in human patients. This is completely rational – few of us would be willing to take a drug or have an implant fitted that might have adverse consequences, which may have been avoided had it been tested on animals – but it is increasingly controversial.

According to statistics provided by the UK Home Office and the United States Department of Agriculture (the governmental agencies that oversee the use of animals in research in the UK and United States respectively), in 2016 3,530 dogs were used in biomedical experiments in the UK and 60,979 in the United States. I fully understand the need for regulating these new therapies, and the intent of the regulations controlling this work is closely scrutinised by governments on both sides of the Atlantic. Furthermore, there are many initiatives, such as the UK-based National Centre for the Replacement, Refinement and Reduction of Animals in Research (NC3Rs), to reduce the number of animals used in these sorts of studies. Great efforts are being made to replace animal tests with non-animal alternatives, such as cell culture experiments and even computer models, as I've already illustrated having enrolled as an experimental model myself in Ohio for spinal research. The good news is that these initiatives appear to be making some inroads – the most recent figures published show that between 2016 and 2017, the number of dogs used in experiments in the UK had fallen by almost 50 per cent.

A complete ban on animal testing seems an unrealistic expectation at this point in time; there is too much at stake, and there is currently a paucity of validated non-animal test alternatives for assessing the safety of new drugs and medical devices for human use. What I would like to focus on is the middle ground: a scenario in which animals, humans and the developers of new drugs or implants might all benefit. The answer lies in leveraging knowledge gained from conscientiously treating the clinical patients that are seen in veterinary practices like mine every day while genuinely helping these animals – dogs, cats and other species – with serious medical conditions, and caring families looking for answers, treatments and hope.

I have sometimes received generous praise for performing first-of-their-kind surgical procedures in dogs, even though I know that the success of these procedures has often been built on a foundation of knowledge from animals who have previously helped advances in the human medical field. As an example, Suzie and her mum came to me from Aberdeenshire in October 2010, after being told by several other veterinary centres that total shoulder replacement was not possible in dogs. In fact, a scientific paper published in 1946 demonstrated successful shoulder replacement in experimental dogs that were then used as models for human joint replacement. It was, therefore, rather embarrassing and indeed nonsensical for me to receive praise for doing something that had been possible for more than sixty years! I have been using customised implants in animals for more than a decade and have always been prepared to share my results with colleagues in human medicine. The advent of additive manufacturing – three-dimensional printing – has revolutionised the process of developing custom implants in humans and animals, and it would be tremendous to think that lessons learned in both human and animal surgery might one day inform progress for both fields in tandem. A middle ground would involve learning from what people like me may already know, so that we can perhaps reduce the need for reliance on experimental animals to inform progress in human surgery.

For the first time in medical history, it is now possible to obtain high-definition scans and to use special software to look in detail at the junction (interface) between bone and a metal implant, as I've alluded to already. For an amputation prosthesis, like that used in Mitzi, we do not need to perform a study in a healthy research dog to determine the effects of the implant on the bone – we can instead monitor the response in a clinical patient who will benefit from the implant. In a similar vein, we now have access to sophisticated laboratory tests to track the behaviour of naturally occurring cancers in veterinary clinical animals (in other words, animals – dogs, cats and even horses – brought into a veterinary surgery for treatment of their illness). Animals with various cancers (neoplasia), ranging from bone cancer to lymphoma to bladder cancer and brain cancer, can now be enrolled in ethically robust clinical trials if the families of those animals so wish.

Some new therapies that may be available are still experimental, in that their effectiveness is unknown, but are given with every expectation that they might slow or prevent the progression of the disease, improve quality of life and perhaps even extend the lives of these companion animals. The results from these clinical trials – some of which are being conducted right now in clinics around the globe within the framework of very strict ethical vigilance and fully informed volitional consent of families – have the potential to save the lives of both animals and humans, without the need to sacrifice a healthy animal's life in the quest for this new knowledge.

For all of these reasons, it makes sense to think of clinical trials in veterinary cancer patients as an important, and currently undervalued, bridge to clinical trials in human patients. By linking a veterinary clinical trial to a human drug development pipeline, we leverage the sort of financial resources that would simply not be possible for 'just' a veterinary drug.

In other words, animals will not get these drugs for a very long time without such cooperation, because the human drug market is far bigger and more lucrative, and there is a lack of money in veterinary medicine to fund trials just to treat cancer in dogs and cats. Pharmaceutical companies could potentially save money by developing drugs in this way, and importantly make new drugs – which may be much better than what we now have – available in dramatically shorter timeframes for both humans and animals. Right now, it can take several years to get any promising new drug from an ex-perimental animal model actually into clinical patients, who often die before the drug becomes available. Furthermore, many drugs showing promise in laboratory settings fail in clinical trials in naturally occurring cancer, and at least some of this attrition of financial resource and loss of animal life could be stemmed by a new framework of collaboration.

I firmly believe that for the first time in history a revo-lution is now possible, if clinical animal and clinical human medical practice worked together. Until now a true two-way street of One Medicine hasn't been possible.

To take an example, carboplatin is a platinum-based drug that is a frontline treatment for bone cancer (osteosarcoma) in both humans and dogs. It is also used in patients with some ovarian and lung cancers. Carboplatin was patented in 1972, and first marketed widely in the UK in the late 1980s. We could probably have a better drug to use, but development is painstakingly slow and incredibly expensive. Results obtained in mouse models of osteosarcoma may not accurately predict the response of the tumour (or the mouse) to a new drug. In contrast, if we take a sample of tumour from a dog with osteosarcoma and have it examined under a microscope by veterinary and human pathologists, they would be hard-pushed to tell whether the sample came from human or canine. The biology of the disease is extremely similar in the two species, and these similarities continue all the way down to the level of genetic mutations within the cancer cells themselves. Osteosarcoma in dogs represents a very relevant model of the disease in humans. Furthermore, the lifespan of the cancer and the dog is shorter than for humans and so clinical trials are therefore more rapidly achieved. I lose patients with bone cancer every month and I dearly wish that I had a better treatment for them. Collaborations between doctors, veterinarians and scientists will undoubtedly identify targets for new drugs to treat tumours in both species. It makes no sense to me whatsoever to not cooporate for the greater good.

In my view, we desperately need to develop a framework in which new therapies can be evaluated systematically and ethically in veterinary patients. Strict ethical governance would of course protect against testing experimental drugs or implants made from entirely untested materials. There would be a requirement for these therapies to have undergone preliminary screening to demonstrate that they do not pose an unacceptable risk in terms of toxicity, but they would potentially not need to have been tested in an artificial model of the disease, resulting in the death of an animal, when a naturally occurring version occurs daily in much-loved family dogs, for which decades-old drugs are still being used in clinical practice. The results from well-designed and carefully regulated veterinary clinical trials can feed directly into the knowledge database and provide critical support for proposed clinical trials in humans. By sharing knowledge, we will be able to change lives; to improve them, to extend them, to protect them – the fundamental tenets of being a medical or veterinary professional. It is this melding of human and animal health into a single scientific endeavour – beyond anything else – that now drives me.

This concept is not new. In the late 1800s, the father of modern pathology, Rudolf Virchow, stated: 'Between animal and human medicine there are no dividing lines – nor should there be.' The term 'One Medicine' was first used by American veterinarian Calvin W. Schwabe in 1984. Since then, the collaboration of veterinarians and human doctors has become known as 'One Health'. To my mind, the challenge is that the current One Health model tends to see humans as the beneficiaries of advances in animal health. Wouldn't it be better to have a One Medicine that sets out to help both humans and animals equally, and not at the expense of an animal life? I am specifically referring here to a concept of One Medicine that truly helps animals as well as humans, not a model of One Health that primarily still focuses on gains that can be achieved for humans through the use of an animal model, which just *might* help animals. The endeavour I'm firmly focused on *must* help animals affected by real disease and must not sacrifice an animal life in the process.

Studying naturally occurring disease in veterinary clinical patients has important advantages with regard to the clinical relevance of our findings. Clinical patients tend to be in their home environment, they are exposed to the sorts of environmental factors that human patients experience, including potential inducers of cancer (carcinogens), and they are cared for and loved in a way that is more typical of human patients. Evaluating these treatments in our patients could be very cost-efficient for the developer of a new drug, since there are no experimental animals to purchase and house in a laboratory; and for cancers that are common in dogs, results can be obtained relatively quickly. Older dogs and cats often have multiple medical conditions – perhaps heart disease in addition to the arthritis that causes them to limp – and this makes them much more relevant as models for human patients, who often have multiple concurrent health complaints. With fully informed family consent, we can potentially make use of blood samples collected from routine check-ups and follow the response to treatment over much longer periods than is possible or affordable for an experimental model in research animals.

There are, of course, significant scientific challenges associated with studying companion animals with naturally occurring diseases as subjects in clinical trials. One of the most problematic relates to how we determine the safety of a drug or an implant. When 'terminal' studies are performed in research animals, the animal is given a standardised treatment and evaluated over a defined time period. At the end of the study, the animal is killed and lots of different tissues are sent to the pathologist for microscopic examination. The results represent a very robust test of safety. In veterinary clinical trials, we are much more limited in terms of what we can do. In the UK, most veterinary clinical trials have to be performed using procedures that are consistent with what is known as 'recognised veterinary practice'. This means that we can only perform procedures that are routinely used in the management of animals with a particular disorder. Everything a veterinary surgeon can do must be in the direct interest of the animal, with disclosure of all other options to the guardians of that animal. We cannot take additional blood samples, we cannot collect tissues from around the implant (unless there is a clinical need to go back in and do a second surgery), and we can only obtain tissues from animals after they die, either from their disease or from natural causes. In my experience, however, at the natural end of life of a family dog or cat, most families will recognise that we have done our best to reduce suffering and prolong the life of their friend, and so they often wish to help other animals and humans in the future by allowing a post mortem examination. It's also important to recognise that there is a second route to performing veterinary clinical trials, but this involves Home Office approval for more invasive procedures. Very few centres in the UK have this capability and approval is challenging to obtain, particularly in a clinical veterinary environment, and may also carry reputational and institutional risk with regard to public perception of such a scenario. Many perceptions and governance issues will need to be addressed if a true two-way street of One Medicine is to be realised in clinical veterinary practice to help animals actually affected by disease in a potentially more expedient and efficacious fashion.

There are also ethical and moral dilemmas with this approach. Even with appropriate oversight from regulatory bodies, there is the potential for side effects that could make the drug or implant less effective than current alternatives. This could possibly disincentivise both the families of animals (in case it could harm their animal friend), and pharmaceutical companies (in case it could prejudice a possible human clinical trial). How should we balance our drive for new knowledge against the fact that we cannot always be sure that a treatment is safe in a given patient? These are questions that will need to be resolved, but I remain convinced that if there is good evidence demonstrating the safety of the drug in cell culture experiments (and perhaps rodent models have already been explored anyway), then it could become possible to move more quickly to veterinary clinical patients. Do we really live in a society where this is deemed less acceptable than studying an artificial form of the disease induced in healthy dogs, cats or other species? This is a fundamental choice for society to make – I am merely shining a light to bring the issue into much-needed sharp focus. Somehow drug development times and expense need to be reduced, without compromising safety. In my opinion, this could be achieved if we made better use of a One Medicine approach in which appropriately regulated veterinary clinical trials provide the families of sick or injured animals an opportunity to consent to advances in medical therapy which may benefit their animal friend, while at the same time contributing to new knowledge that will impact both human and animal health.

In my opinion, the current status quo – one in which healthy animals are used as a walking test tube, with no real emphasis on using the results of these studies to improve animal health – needs to change. It seems an undeniable truth that until computer models and non-animal alternatives are fully validated, there will remain a need for some degree of preclinical safety testing in animals for human drugs and implants, but we need to alter the way that drugs and devices are evaluated from that point on. If companion animals have diseases that mirror those seen in humans, there should be no need to artificially induce the disease in healthy animals. Drug and implant companies can make the same amount of money, or more, by working alongside veterinarians like myself who are discovering the answers to many of the questions that would otherwise need to be addressed by terminal studies in research animals.

As with the gradual progress with limb amputation prostheses in Storm, Coal, Oscar and Mitzi, I am not of the view that everything can, or indeed should, change overnight, but I do firmly believe that if we change a little day by day, if we respect animals more, then medicine will generally change for the better, society will become more compassionate and both animals and humans will win in the end. Put simply, we cannot expect a different outcome if we continue to do the same thing. In my lifetime, I will do all I can to prompt a significant paradigm shift for pharmaceutical and implant companies and for regulatory bodies so that animals get a fairer deal as time goes by. This idea is at the heart of everything I've striven for throughout my career: respect for animals and the advancement of veterinary and human medicine side by side.

To achieve these twin goals, in 2010, I was determined to found a charity to stand up for animals and also to secure another television deal on which I could continue to build a platform for awareness that the love between a human and an animal can and should translate into a broader responsibility for animals everywhere. If we had the same bond of love for a rhinoceros or an elephant as we do companion animals, would we be facing extinction of so many beautiful species right now?

Despite its popularity, *The Bionic Vet*, broadcast in 2010, wasn't recommissioned, and while patients like Mitzi and Suzie kept the flame burning inside me, getting another TV show commissioned was proving more challenging than I had hoped. Throughout 2011 and into 2012, I emailed everyone

I could find online who might be interested in such a series, but I couldn't get a meeting with any of them. I knew in my heart that the idea was viable, but getting a commission wasn't dependent on how hard I worked, it was about who I could get in front of, and that required luck, serendipity and a modicum of charm, rather than hard graft and surgical ability.

The Bionic Vet had helped shape the thoughts that were forming in my head about what might come next, but I had a practice to run, patients to treat, clients to serve, a growing team to pay and a bank loan to service, so I hunkered down to work. That didn't mean I stopped trying to get another TV show off the ground, though. I must have pitched the idea that ultimately became *The Supervet* a couple of dozen times before finally, in early 2012, a producer called Steve Hodges, who had come across *The Bionic Vet* and some publicity I had done for it, emailed me to see if I might be interested in a meeting. He recommended that I meet with his co-producer in the States, Vincent DeSalvo. So, in April 2012, when I was flying to America to give lectures, I decided to take a detour to LA to meet DeSalvo.

Could this possibly be the big break I was looking for? I knew I was going to be nervous, so I thought that the best way to conquer that fear was to distract myself by following in the footsteps of one of my personal heroes, who'd also had a particularly stressful time in LA, although for different reasons. I'm a huge Depeche Mode fan, and the songs 'Personal Jesus' and 'Walking in My Shoes' really resonate with me. I knew that Dave Gahan, the lead singer, had been a wild boy and, in 1996, had taken a speedball at the Sunset Marquis Hotel, which stopped his heart and nearly killed him. My critical meeting was taking place in LA and I was determined to stay at the Sunset Marquis: if Dave could survive his trauma, then so could I, even if fear stopped my heart.

I arrived at the hotel and sat in the reception for quite a while, with the intention of finding the oldest concierge that I could. Finally, I saw a likely candidate and approached him in a quiet moment, saying something like, 'Excuse me, please.' He looked at me for a moment, before concluding, '*Oh, you're Irish!*' I didn't need to speak further. It turned out my nationality was my in! He was himself of Irish heritage and we chatted for a while before I finally asked the question, the reason I was here: was there any way at all that he might know the room in which Depeche Mode's Dave Gahan had nearly killed himself? I knew that it was a long shot and I also acknowledge that this fellow could have told me anything and I would've believed him at the time. He could have been selling me a red herring, but he appeared a most genuine and pleasant man, so when he said yes, to my mind he came up trumps. Approaching reception, he asked if that particular room was available. And yet again, my luck, it appeared, was in. I tipped my new friend, let myself into said room and lay down on the bed. I didn't get any major vibe from it and the walls did not emit energies of past guests, but it was still a comforting feeling just to be there. Was it Dave's room? I believed – and still choose to believe to this day – that it was.

A couple of days later, I pitched the first version of *The Supervet* in that very same room and I did a screen test on the balcony, surrounded by palm trees. Despite my best efforts, I tripped over my words, didn't explain concepts well enough and delivered, at best, a mediocre performance. I was dispirited, discouraged and crestfallen. After the production team left, I sat on the bed and heard the voices of my old friends, Philip and Malcolm, in my head, the former gently saying, 'Shall we do that again, do you think?', and Malcolm adding, 'Without the pole up your arse this time!' I'd been so wooden in the audition.

While there, I reached out to another producer who was a friend of a friend and was duly invited to his home in Beverly Hills. I got in the cab, amazed by the opulence of my surroundings as we drove between the beautifully manicured hedges, past palatial properties as the driver pointed out various celebrities' houses. Finally, he pulled over, dropping me outside my apparent destination. I pressed the buzzer, announced my name and was admitted. Walking up the driveway, I came to an imposing mansion where I was greeted with a glass of rather wonderful champagne, before being ushered through the hallway to the back of the ornate house, where a pool party seemed to be in full swing.

Knowing nobody, I sidled up to the bar and sat down. This was a long way from a farm in the bog, kneeling in cow shite while pulling out calves, I mused. While my jaw was hanging open, probably somewhere close to my toes, a rather elegant lady, with very taut facial features and hair coiffed in a most delightful fashion, sat down beside me. We began to chat, at first rather hesitantly on my part, but my Irish brogue seemed to intrigue her. The champagne began to work its magic, as did the sparkle of the pool and of the various glitzy dresses shimmering in the LA sunshine, and soon we were both laughing and joking like old friends. Finally, she asked me how I knew Danny.

Danny? I didn't know any Danny. I was puzzled. That wasn't the name of the guy I was supposed to meet. Confused, I hesitated. She gestured over towards the pool. Standing there in resplendent joviality was a man I immediately recognised, just as she asked me again, 'So, how do you know Danny DeVito?'

Shit! I was at the wrong house! I immediately panicked at the thought of being found out and forcibly expelled, so I just mumbled something incomprehensible about the movie *Twins* and beat a hasty retreat back onto the street. In retrospect, I should have blagged it and seen how I got on, especially as I have since learned that Danny loves dogs and therefore might have helped me out, but a sense of honesty and trepidation swept over me. I called the number I had been given, and with some directing found the right house nearby and met with the actual producer. Sadly, though, it was a wasted journey: I went back home to the UK and to the practice and didn't hear a word. Dejected, but not defeated, I flung myself back into the maelstrom of the surgery and the building works.

Much later, in early 2013, I decided to take matters into my own hands – perhaps in a moment of throwing caution to the wind, considering the pressure I was under because of the forthcoming specialist exams. I concluded that it might be best to create the format for the show myself on camera, so that I could better translate to a production company or a broadcaster what, until that point, had just been inside my head. When my old friend, director-cameraman Jim Incledon, who I had worked with on both *Wildlife SOS* and *The Bionic Vet*, finished one of his many projects and became available, I asked him to help me make a new TV pilot. I bought a RED high-definition television camera and he set up camp at the practice.

Jim followed me around the surgery as I went about my day. I was very comfortable with his presence because we'd been around each other so much in the past. I got on with my own work while he magically captured what I was doing on camera. Jim is a genius in his chosen profession, and he happened to be on the prep-room floor when poor Tiger suffered a cardiac arrest, and was ultimately resuscitated with my finger pumping his heart inside his chest cavity. Jim filmed everything that happened that day, and on many others – real moments of life and death, heartfelt emotions, dilemmas, tragedies and moments of epiphany. He edited together the best of the footage he had shot – and, by May 2013, we knew we had something special to show a production company or broadcaster.

I was immersed in exam fever, as well as operating and running the practice, so I had intended to put the footage to one side until after the UK and US exams were done and then see what could be done with it. What I did not know was that my screen test on that balcony of the Sunset Marquis hadn't been totally in vain. Steve Hodges, the producer who'd originally contacted me early in 2012, had at some point reached out to Nick Hornby, a commissioning editor in Factual Entertainment and Features at Channel 4 and, towards the end of May 2013, Nick and Steve spoke with me by phone.

I pitched my idea for the show after which Nick asked me to come to see him. I suggested that it might be more useful if he could come and see me at the practice instead. He probably thought this cheeky, but I knew that if I could get him into the actual environment to see the families and animals, and just experience the general atmosphere of the place, he might more readily recognise the veterinary programme's potential and audience. Miraculously, he agreed.

When Nick arrived, Jim and I brought him into the lecture theatre at the practice. As we sat down to show him some of the footage we had filmed, including the story of Tiger, I could hear my daddy, as we sheltered from the rain in the hay barn, all those years ago, telling me to keep my cool and reminding me that 'strength of mind is more powerful than strength of the body'. Nick said nothing throughout the film, but his total concentration and focus gave me great hope. It turned out that he was impressed and a door had opened for us. Jim and I were finally in with a chance to share the rest of our vision, and I'm forever grateful to him for sticking by my side. A few weeks later, Nick emailed me to say that he was debating the best place for the programme, 'because', as he wrote, 'it's so unlike what the public would imagine a standard documentary about pets and vets would be like'.

My understanding is that Channel 4 then explored potential partners with which to make the proposed show, at the time given the working title *Animal ER*. Steve Hodge's production company was in that mix, as was Blast, the production company that finally ended up making the programme. I personally feel sad for Steve Hodges, as it was his initial interest that led to the breakthrough that Jim and I needed following the making of the pilot, but I suppose that's how life is sometimes.

I find the business side of making television quite difficult, in that it requires a big team of people, just like Fitzpatrick Referrals, and it carries with it different specific logistical and financial demands for the production company. Without Jim, there is no doubt that *The Supervet* would never have existed, and because he and I had already created most of the footage on our own for the first episodes, long before Blast came on board, it still amazes me how complex the 'machinery' of making television becomes in order to actually have a programme successfully broadcast.

The show wasn't formally commissioned until later in 2013, however, when Jay Hunt approved it. Jay had also commissioned *The Bionic Vet,* and had moved from the BBC to become the head of Channel 4. Needless to say, the programme would probably never have seen the light of day there had Jay not still believed in me, for which I'm very grateful. During that time, there was much discussion about a suitable programme title. In my mind, it boiled down to calling it *The Bionic Vet* again or my proposed personal favourite, *The Supervet.* The former wasn't appetising enough for the broadcaster and the title had already changed from *Animal ER* to *24/7 Animal Surgery.* They were still considering a dozen or so other possible working titles, before they finally went with *The Supervet.* Suddenly my dream was a reality and it seemed my team and I were about to embark on our most exciting and most challenging journey yet.

The first episode of our new TV show aired on 7 May 2014. Making *The Supervet* has been a challenge, as it takes considerable time and effort. Because I had already made *The Bionic Vet*, I was used to having cameramen around so that aspect wasn't initially problematic, but once there were fixed-rig cameras on the walls in different departments of the practice, it became a whole new version of reality for the team and myself. It was hard for everyone to get used to having the cameras on all the time, but everyone at Fitzpatrick Referrals embraced it, knowing that it was for an important reason, bigger than all of us.

In fact, without television, my wonderful surgical resident, Padraig Egan, a popular member of the Fitz-family and frequent contributor to *The Supervet*, would never have even come to Fitzpatrick Referrals as an intern. He emailed me, after having seen an episode of *The Bionic Vet*, and I replied to him that same night around midnight. I hired him a week later. In early 2019, Padraig will take his specialist exams, after his surgical residency training at Fitzpatrick Referrals. I'm very happy for him and proud for our practice.

The power of the message one can deliver on television is profound. Of course, as with *The Bionic Vet*, there must be trust between my colleagues, the families who allow us to travel their journeys with them and the production team. The families have selflessly allowed people throughout the world to see them in very vulnerable times of crisis with their ill and injured beloved animal friends and my colleagues at Fitzpatrick Referrals work under the spotlight of the camera almost daily. The production team don't get any opportunities for 'retakes' since this is real life. My gratitude to each and every one of these people is heartfelt and boundless. It is an undeniable fact that the participating families have, in four short years, done more to change perceptions about veterinary medicine and the importance of respect for animals than I have done in my entire lifetime outside of the TV show.

The Supervet is helping to communicate that animals really are integral family members, that they deserve a fair deal and that, for the first time in the history of veterinary medicine, medical techniques are moving forward at the same speed, or even faster, than in human medicine. Viewers everywhere are aware of this revolution and, as I have said before in this book, once one knows something is possible, it's impossible not to know that it's possible. My hope is that this will over time translate into real and tangible progress with regard to respect for animals and the medical advances they deserve.

I think that Channel 4 wondered just how the public would

receive this new kind of animal hospital show when it was first broadcast, however. It wasn't quite science, nor did it adhere to the previous formula of veterinary programming. It was something completely new. By the end of 2018, when this book is published, series twelve and over eighty episodes will have aired in the UK, which gives me hope that there is a general will to respect and rejoice in the human–animal bond. I think the show resonates with people because we're searching for compassion in a world which can be crazy, and in which there can be a vacuum where bad thoughts and actions sometimes grow, where often sometimes we don't know what to believe and where people's inhumanity to each other can sometimes leave us empty and sad. The love of an animal is something real that we can all relate to regardless of colour, creed, sexuality or religion. Dogs and cats don't care about such things – they love us and we love them back (well, most of us) unconditionally – and I think that's important, in a world sometimes consumed with superficial, seemingly unimportant things.

Like anything in the public arena, *The Supervet* gets negative as well as positive reviews. However, thankfully, the balance is generally tipped in favour of the latter. Members of the public have generally been supportive and generous, like the big guy covered in tattoos who, one night in a restaurant, gave me a nudge and said, 'All right, Noel, thanks for looking after the dogs', and the lady in the street who stopped me and gave me a big hug, and the disabled man who loves the show and went to a print shop to have three dogs printed on a couple of hoodies, one for himself and one for me, above the caption: 'Money can buy you things, but it doesn't lick your face and wag its tail every time it sees you.' All of these kindnesses seem possible because of the TV show – and I think that generally the world is better for that.

There are downsides, of course – such as being recognised all the time. One such occasion was when I was knackered after an event I founded called Dogfest, a festival where everyone who loves a dog can join with like-minded folks in a giant field to make friends and give dogs their best possible day out, with activities for all ages. I was driving home and stopped at a motorway service station to make a rather urgent call of nature. I parked hurriedly and made a dash for the public toilet, pulling up my hoodie for fear of being recognised by people who might inevitably be driving back from Dogfest – and in that particular moment I had a very specific desire to get where I was going very quickly indeed. I kept walking, head down along the long and winding route that aims to entice one to buy things one doesn't really need. With a great sense of relief, I got as far as the sinks and turned around to find a toilet cubicle I most certainly did need by that point. Unfortunately, as I pulled down my hood, I was greeted by the excited shrieks of a little girl hollering loudly, 'Hey everybody! It's The Supervet!' It was only then that I realised that I had inadvertently rushed into the ladies! I shall write the headline for the tabloids now – '*Supervet Found in Ladies' Toilets on the M6!*'

The positives of making the programme far outweigh any negatives, though, and the show has opened doors that would have been otherwise impossible even to kick down. By far the most important has been the opportunity to finally found the charity I had in my heart for many years, The Humanimal Trust, which funds education and research, advancing medical knowledge for animals and humans in tandem, but *never* at the expense of an animal life. It's a true two-way street of One Medicine. As I have said in so many ways, it has long been my dream that the existing dichotomy between human and veterinary medicine might be addressed by building a platform where human and veterinary medical professionals, researchers and scientists learn from each other, and where animals that need solutions who, in other circumstances, might have been put to sleep, may go on, instead, to live longer and happier lives. This in turn informs progress in medical science in a way that might help every species. The Humanimal Trust charity embodies my life's purpose and my legacy. It is the single most important endeavour of my life.

Without *The Supervet*, the trustees and I would not have been able to raise enough of a profile to achieve funding for the first few projects we have sponsored, and without Fitzpatrick Referrals, the charity would never have happened at all.

A black Labrador, called Kariba, walked into my consulting room, with her dad, David Hart, in December 2013. She had developmental elbow disease. David subsequently helped me and my colleague, Dineke Abbing, to convert my existing educational vehicle, the Fitzpatrick Education Foundation, into The Humanimal Trust – humans and animals trusting each other for the greater good. Although we have a very long way to go, with The Humanimal Trust we have put a flagpole in the ground for One Medicine. I fully intend to wave this flag until my dying day.

Just a few years ago, it did not seem likely that I would get a TV show commissioned, let alone that it would be successful, or that I would be able to found The Humanimal Trust. From an early age, I have believed with all of my heart in One Medicine, even though I didn't know what it was called when I was a child looking at my own bruises as I fell from the chestnut tree, or while watching Daddy mend a lamb's leg and drawing parallels in my head, or looking with horror at Uncle Paul's sore amputation stump and wondering why he and Vetman's hedgehog couldn't both have bionic legs. Through the years, everything that I have done – all the education I have sought, every academic, professional and media endeavour I have undertaken – has been in some way directed towards my life goal of unifying animal and human medicine in mutual respect and compassion. The odds were stacked against all of the achievements to date, but they have happened.

I wonder how many of those who've watched *The Supervet* have seen the chestnut tree in the hedgerow side by side with the cherry blossom tree that I planted for my dear friends Philip and Malcolm, to remind me to 'always do the right thing, even when nobody is watching', and to always believe in my reason big enough. An aerial view of the practice is shown in almost all episodes of *The Supervet*, and yet I would guess maybe the odds are stacked against any viewer ever having recognised these trees. The most important physical representations of everything that is important to me is in plain sight, yet it is these things that most don't see.

Very sadly, shortly after I had planted it at our practice in Eashing, the chestnut tree got blown down in a big storm in 2008. It had snapped off at the base of the trunk, disease attacked the roots and it had visibly died. I was devastated and thought I had lost forever that last tangible link to my friend Philip, the man who had inspired me to chase the field of dreams in the first place, and the tree that I looked at every day to give me hope, even in my darkest hour. His memory had lived on for me in the emerging branches of that chestnut, just like the one I had climbed as a child, stretching outwards with its five-fingered leaves.

Several months after her operation, Mitzi the white German shepherd dog was out in the field behind the practice, and I was throwing sticks for her, testing her recovery as she sped around, twisting and turning on her bionic foot, using it as successfully as if it was actually part of her own body. I absentmindedly reached into the hedgerow nearby and snapped off a bit of a sapling to throw for her and, as she brought it back to me, I realised that it was a sprig of chestnut tree. I looked in the undergrowth, and to my astonishment found that the base of Philip's tree was growing again. It hadn't died after all, and hope lived on – nature's miraculous capacity to regenerate in both a dog and a tree. The chances of Mitzi being in that field at that time, with her bionic foot, and leading me to the rediscovery of Philip's tree were extraordinarily unlikely, but against all of the odds, it happened.

I smiled to myself, and thanked Philip for the important reminder that my reason big enough is still rooted with me in the soil of Fitzpatrick Referrals.

CHAPTER EIGHTEEN

Willow

The Currency of Love

I am profoundly grateful that *The Supervet* gives me an amazing platform to show the real-life journey of love and hope for people who deeply care about animals, and in so doing engenders greater respect for animals and explores the possibility of medical and surgical solutions where none previously existed. I also hope that the acknowledgement of an animal as an integral family member will in time translate to a broader responsibility for all animals globally, both domestic and wild. But the day-to-day reality of trying to achieve this is no bed of roses.

I find 'living in the public eye' really difficult even though I've chosen to place myself on television. I accept that this makes me fair game for social media commentary, but sometimes the attempted character assassination is very wounding. If, despite every best effort, a procedure goes wrong or a treatment fails, families can sometimes become very angry and even accusatory. In general, however, the negative or derogatory comments aimed at me are from people or organisations with different opinions or agendas, and very sadly for me this includes fellow veterinary professionals. They are entitled to their opinion, and all I can do is encourage them to try to realise that fundamentally I think we all want the same thing: a better world for animals and for our families to live in and to inherit. Unfortunately, I do take it all very personally, and though misguided hostility will not derail me from my mission, I would be lying if I said that the criticism doesn't sometimes really hurt.

Soon after we had started filming *The Supervet* in 2014, one Thursday night at around 10 p.m., I sat by the computer in my consulting room with my head in my hands, beyond worn out. We had seen patients all day, and I had just come out of my fifth surgery, a particularly gruelling one. I have felt exhausted many times over the past twenty-five years of practice life, but somehow this time it was different. It was tiredness mixed with a sense of foreboding. I knew my next case was going to be bad as soon as I had spoken to the referring vet.

I flicked on the lights in my consulting room, as the limp, skinny body of a two-year-old lurcher called Willow was carried in, accompanied by her family, Noreen, Graham and eleven-year-old Lev. Before I'd come out of my previous operation, my clinical team and the TV production assistant had asked permission for the cameras to be running. The family consented, wanting to help both Willow and any other dog in the future as best they could.

The young dog had run into a tree and broken her neck and now lay motionless on a rug on my floor, whimpering; she was in extreme pain, her neck strained backwards, her eyes wide open and bloodshot with fear. She had lost the ability to move any of her limbs and seemed to just about feel it when I pinched her toes. She was paralysed – or, to be more precise, non-ambulatory tetraparetic. It was a life-or-death situation and it was clear that we had to make a decision over how to proceed urgently – to put her down or try to operate. Was it better to try to save her or just let Willow slip peacefully away? Noreen, Graham and Lev were all in bits. The young boy just sat there staring at his hands, in obvious turmoil. Their thoughts hung heavily on the air; the atmosphere was beyond tense. The silence as I examined her could only have lasted for a moment, but seemed like an eternity. She was deteriorating in front of our eyes, and in significant pain.

I quickly and quietly explained that if we were to put Willow through surgery, there would be massive risks and it would be very tough. I said that while there was a chance she might run around again, this was by no means a certainty. Noreen and Graham asked if I could scan Willow's spine to see just how serious the fracture was and I explained that it wasn't always possible to see just how badly the cord was damaged and that it wouldn't establish if an operation would be successful or not. All I could promise to do was our best under these circumstances. After the scan, Noreen, Graham and Lev would have a very difficult decision to make. They went into the waiting room, clinging onto each other and the last vestiges of hope.

With Willow now anaesthetised, the team I went to the scanner, our hearts in our mouths, Willow's life in our hands. The scan only took a few seconds, but the couple of minutes for the reconstruction of the images seemed to drag like a rope of barbed wire in my head. We found that Willow had suffered a comminuted mid-body fracture of the second cervical vertebra (the axis – which I call the 'no' bone as we shake our head on it) just behind the first cervical vertebra (the atlas – which I call the 'yes' bone since we nod on it). In other words she had a very bad broken neck, the break just behind the point at which the spinal cord comes off the back of the brain. The spinal cord had been severely damaged by pressure from the displaced vertebrae and pieces of shattered bone that poked into it like spears. The bony prominence at the front of the axis (the 'dens'), on which the atlas rotates, was also sticking up into the spinal cord as the two vertebrae had been pummelled together and forcibly torn apart by the impact when she hit the tree.

This was a worst possible case fracture scenario because the bone fragments were tiny and I couldn't put pins directly in them – I would have to use the bone on either side to anchor and then pull apart, or distract, the imploded fracture. Furthermore, there was no guarantee that after all this intervention the spinal cord would actually mend – so Willow could go through surgery and still not recover. Most risky of all, though, was the probability that as soon as we moved the broken vertebrae fragments, we would likely get a volcano of uncontrollable bleeding from very thin-walled venous sinuses, which are particularly large in the axis bone, on the base of the spinal canal. These sinuses would almost certainly have been shredded by the impact. As soon as I moved those spiky bits of bone, if I was unlucky and couldn't stem the bleeding, Willow could potentially lose about 5 ml of blood every second if I couldn't get the bones set back together again quickly enough. She most certainly could bleed to death during the surgery. There would be no safe route to get inside the canal to stop the bleeding once the fragments were moved.

I called the family back into the consulting room, the weight of their anxiety and distress now weighing heavily on my shoulders, too. If possible, young Lev was even more ashen than before and Noreen was trembling, as she clutched Graham's hand. Their eyes were full of anguish as I explained the gravity of the situation, then Noreen and I both tried to break it down for Lev. He just nodded. Noreen and Graham stared helplessly at each other.

'Are you OK?' Noreen asked me, her voice breaking the heavy silence in the room. Her question surprised me: no one ever asks me if I am OK. Understandably, the welfare of the surgeon is not normally the foremost concern of the family in a time of extreme crisis. The usual questions after an extreme diagnosis might be, 'What would you do if it were your dog?' or 'Do you think it's best if we allow her to pass away?' On this night, however, it was different, and I was in a very bad mental, emotional and physical state. Noreen caring enough to ask how I was feeling was a very unusual moment.

Noreen's extraordinary compassion pulled down all my barriers, and so in that moment I didn't do what I normally do and just say, 'I'm fine.' I hesitated for a moment, taken aback by her kindness. I am emotionally invested in each and every one of my patients, but in this moment all of my emotions were stripped bare. Noreen's insightful question prompted an unguarded, most personal answer. I said to Graham and Noreen that I was physically exhausted and that I was worried about undertaking such a massively challenging procedure so late into the night. I also explained to them that the surgery was a procedure about which there was little published, not many surgeons had to my knowledge performed it, and that even if we attempted it the outcome was very unpredictable in the circumstances. I reassured them that I would operate if they wanted me to, as long as they understood that even if I did my absolute best, that might not be good enough and we could still fail.

Noreen looked at Graham and together they said that they would like me to try to save Willow. I asked them if they were sure and if they all understood that she may die on the table or thereafter. I reiterated that as soon as I moved the bones I may be unable to stop the bleeding, or I might not be able to get the pins inserted in enough bone to develop adequate traction to pull the spiky fragments down from the spinal canal, or I may not be able to stabilise the bones adequately, among other possible complications. They nodded and signed the consent form.

I gave them each a hug as I said goodbye and told them to try to get some rest, if they could, reassuring them that I'd be in touch as soon as the operation was finished. As little Lev reached up his arms to me, I could feel his fear and his pain acutely and I could also feel him placing all of his hope and trust in me. Noreen had explained off camera that Lev and Willow had formed an extremely close bond, partly, she confided in me, because both of them were adopted. She has since allowed me to share this information. It was obvious how much Lev loved Willow, but this imparted a whole new level of responsibility for me going into theatre. At that moment, for me, Noreen being one of the most kind, considerate and insightful women on earth, and caring about Willow, Lev and even me, in the midst of this crisis, was truly extraordinary.

As I stood at the scrub sink I closed my eyes, unconsciously reverting back to when Pirate was my best friend, just like Willow was Lev's. I was about the same age as Lev when I lost those lambs and in that moment I empathised with him feeling scared and helpless, as I recalled lying on that frosty field, looking up at the brightest star in heaven, wishing I was strong enough, brave enough and clever enough to make things better. I could now see that light vividly in my mind's eye as I scrubbed my hands and rocked backwards and forwards at the sink, trying to psych myself up and break through the exhaustion. As I kicked open the door of theatre, the familiar adrenaline surge came and suddenly I was as alert as an astronaut about to land on the moon.

The team was in place – surgery is never a solo effort and the nurses, theatre auxiliaries, radiographer and interns were all as tired as I was, but also as determined to do their utmost to save Willow. She lay on the operating table, the surgical site was sterilised and the surgical field was surrounded by drapes. I cut underneath her neck from just under her jaw bone backwards towards her breast bone. Then I used my fingers to separate the neck muscles and to push the windpipe, the food pipe, the veins, arteries and nerves all over to one side. Slowly, I scraped the muscle off the bottom of the vertebrae and immediately the bleeding started. Even without having moved the bones, blood was already starting to gush through the brittle shattered debris of the vertebrae.

I packed the site temporarily with collagen sponges to stem the bleeding, then set to work figuring out which bits of bone I could pick up with some pins. I carefully drilled the cartilage out of the joint between the atlas and the axis vertebrae so that when the bones were pulled apart and the dens and spiky bits came back down into position, everything could fuse together as one solid block. The damage would not ever allow the atlas and axis to move independently again anyway, and I needed bone in front of the imploded front half of the axis vertebra in which to anchor pins. Gingerly, I placed pins into the atlas bone, so as not to skewer the cord, a perilously tight target, before placing a collection of pins into the remaining back half of the axis vertebra. Then, because I knew there wouldn't be enough purchase for the metal in the bone still remaining in the axis, I also put pins in the third cervical vertebra behind that.

Next, I performed a procedure which reminded me of making moulds for concrete 'silt traps' which my daddy had taught me years ago in the Glebe when we were putting down shores. These traps were cement boxes that punctuated lengths of drainage pipes, so that dirt could drop down and away from the water in the pipes. They were constructed by pouring cement around small planks of wood that were pulled apart by small twigs tied with twine. In this case, I carefully drilled 2 mm-diameter threaded pins into Willow's atlas, the third cervical vertebra and what was left of the back end of the axis on either side of the shattered vertebral body. I bent the ends of the pins over like hooks, under which I threaded wire attached to distraction tools – like Daddy's twigs and twine – so that I could pull the vertebrae apart. Wide wooden lollipop-stick tongue depressors would serve as guidance – like Daddy's planks of wood – on each of the four sides as I poured the bone cement in the middle. However, the trickiest and most dangerous bit was yet to come.

Based on Willow's body weight, I reckoned I'd likely have about three-and-a-half minutes to pull the bones apart, set them in place with the cement around the pins and stop the bleeding before she almost certainly died, either then, or later due to organ failure, in spite of the various fluid drips she was on. I decided that the best chance she had was for me to distract the bones and pour in the liquid cement at the same time to try to stem the bleeding by physically blocking it. I hoped that I could estimate how much to distract before the cement set so as to stretch the fragments back into position: too much and the pins might break or pull out of the bone and all was lost; too little, and the cement would set while the bone fragments were still squashing the spinal cord. I was metaphorically blindfolded because this would all happen beneath the cement while I poured. I had to pour this cement while it was liquid such that it would get into the nooks and crannies before it was moulded using the lollipop sticks, and I had to pull the pins apart before it set. This in itself was an additional challenge. Biological bone cement is a polymer called polymethyl methacrylate, consisting of powder to which a special liquid is added, so it then transforms from very fluid to runny to gloopy to set solid within about five-and-a-half minutes or so (depending on cement type and room temperature).

Bone cement also releases a tremendous amount of heat as it sets rock hard (exothermic curing), so I took bone marrow from Willow's humerus bones, just beneath her shoulders, which has a consistency like sponge cake and, during distraction, had it ready to pack quickly in place, just like grouting, into the drilled-out joint and the gaps between the pieces of shattered bone. The bone marrow graft would ultimately help Willow's bones to heal and simultaneously provide a base for the mould so that the cement wouldn't leak into the cracks or touch the spinal cord and potentially damage the sensitive nerves with its high setting temperature. So, there were just three minutes to distract, pack the graft and pour the cement, and about a minute-and-a-half to shape the cement in the mould before it would rapidly set. Easy!

I pulled the bones apart as far as I dared and the blood started to well up as I'd predicted. On and on it came, bubbling up from the volcano below. I packed the graft as I continued to stretch the pins with their wire nooses apart, and then at just the right moment, I poured and shaped the cement. Holding my breath, I watched as the cement set hard. Finally, with a few last bubbling gasps, the bleeding stopped. I gasped too, finally able to breathe again, as I removed the lollipop planks, trimmed off the pins where they stuck out from the base of the cement, flushed the open wound and stitched Willow up.

Then I waited. A trickle of sweat snaked down my neck as the post-operative radiographs and CT scans came through. I closed my eyes tightly, thinking of the love I had for my own friend Pirate all those years ago as I hugged him and talked to him in times of need, before opening them again. Then a big sigh of relief from both the radiographer and myself – all was well. The fragments were almost perfectly in alignment, Willow's vertebrae were stable and her spinal cord was decompressed. Now it all came down to the ability of her spinal cord to heal.

It was close to 3 a.m. when I was finally able to call Noreen at her home to inform her that Willow was in recovery, attentively watched over by the night nurses. Now, only time would tell. If she could have thrown her arms down the phone line and hugged me, she would have, as she thanked me from the bottom of her heart on behalf of herself, Graham and especially Lev. She again asked me if I was OK and if there was anything she could do for me. It was quite extraordinary. As I closed my eyes to sleep, I smiled as I allowed myself a rare moment to acknowledge how Vetman might be pleased that I had been strong, brave and maybe even clever enough, at least this one time.

When I went down to the wards later that morning, I crept into the compartment where Willow was resting comfortably on a cocktail of happy drugs. To my absolute delight and amazement, she lifted her head and licked my hand. I pinched her toes and she pulled back on all of them and looked up at me as if clearly saying: 'What are you doing, haven't I been through enough? Yes – I can feel that!' That same day, she was up and walking independently. Biology had, indeed, smiled. Nearly forty years after I had lost the lambs, a star had shone for Willow and Lev.

Several weeks later, Willow came back for her follow-up imaging which confirmed that everything had healed in place with full bone bridging between the vertebrae. The operation had been a success and Willow could return to running around – but I hoped she would be much more careful around trees. I was thrilled to see Lev, when he came in with Noreen; he was beaming with smiles. Knowing the full circumstances of the incredible bond between Lev and Willow, and also by then other details about his life, I realised that this young man and I had much more in common than just our relationships with our canine childhood companions. Lev was being mercilessly bullied at school, just as I had been at his age. He called Willow his 'hairy sister', allowing him some respite from loneliness and isolation. By Lev's own admission, Willow 'was a rescue dog and he was a rescue human'.

Lev's experiences touched me deeply. I shared some of my parallel experiences with him and his family, and reassured Lev that he had all the skills to overcome the difficulties he was facing. I talked to him about bullying and how I had survived, saying that he could too. I wanted to give him something that he could keep to remember what we had talked about, and how he had been part of the difficult decision-making that had ultimately saved Willow. I reminded him that he had taken responsibility and shown great courage that night of Willow's accident, and that he was capable of showing the same courage in facing up to any bully, anytime. I told him that bullies are people who cannot look in the mirror, so they deflect all of their own inadequacy on people like us. I told Lev about Vetman and that he had a special name for a bully – The Man With No Name – because such a human doesn't deserve a name. I gave him my stethoscope so he could always 'listen to the animals', even in his darkest hour. He gave me a big hug, which, for me, was the physical manifestation of why I do what I do.

Vets carry a set of scales in their hearts and heads at all times and try to balance them fairly. When I graduated, there would have been no question whatsoever about Willow's treatment – I would have had to say how sorry I was, but that 'nothing could be done' and sent her on her way. But, now that so many more surgical procedures are possible, that choice does carry with it a greater moral responsibility, both for the vet and for the animal's family, opening up all kinds of questions. Should they proceed with surgery simply because they can? Should they feel bad if they don't? These are difficult dilemmas and we don't always know the answers, but as the veterinary landscape of possibility changes, so, too, does the weighting applied to each side of the scales, and we must balance wisely. Just because it is possible to do something, doesn't necessarily make it the right thing to do, and each particular set of circumstances must be independently considered.

Vets are trained to think rationally, and to make objective judgements, but as I have said before, 'people do not care what you know, until they know that you care'. I think that it's really important that veterinary professionals are emotionally invested and actually feel a type of love for their patients. It can be considered an unnecessary indulgence to talk about love as a concept in veterinary or human medicine and yet it's often the very reason many people decide to go into any medical profession in the first place. Far from being an indulgence, I believe that it is an essential quality. When we deeply care about – that is, *love* – our patients, they give back way more than we could ever possibly give to them, just as Willow did for me on that night in 2014. Somehow, in doing what needs to be done, in loving animals within one's vocation, even above concerns for one's own personal needs, I truly believe there comes peace, there comes redemption. I know that animals have saved me from myself more times than I can recall.

Finally, in 2018, years after Willow's procedure, the technique for fixing her spine has been published and hopefully this in turn will benefit other animals. That said, of all the many academic papers I've tried to get published, I am extremely proud of one, also from 2018, which I co-authored with an ethicist called Anne Gallagher. In fact, 'Towards a humanimal clinical ethics', as it is called, echoes the very ethos of the charity I have founded, The Humanimal Trust. It's one of the few papers dealing with the value of love in a professional medical environment. I believe that the love of an animal can make us the very best we can be and, as I have said, I want to give animals a fair deal and I want the love that we feel for any animal who is part of a family to shine like that brightest star in heaven which shaped my life on that fateful night all those years ago in 1978.

One New Year's Eve, long after I had operated on Willow, I was emotionally at rock bottom. It was one of the worst times of my life because of a broken personal relationship and my heart was shattered. I had lost a woman I loved because I was working all the time and had given my life to the animals, for better or for worse, on days and nights when I could, and maybe should have made different choices. This is so hard, not just for me, but for anyone who doesn't have a job with fixed hours or who has dedicated their life to their vocation. I decided, just before midnight for no apparent reason, to contact Noreen. I just wanted to talk to someone and there wasn't anyone else so I emailed a virtual stranger who had once brought a magnificent light into my life when I really needed it. I thanked her and Graham for bringing Willow and Lev into my life because this light was helping me now when I needed it more than ever. I thought maybe I was just writing into the darkness of the universe, and didn't realistically expect a reply.

At four minutes to midnight, Noreen replied. She said that Willow had a wonderful life now, secure, loved and joyfully running free through the woods near their home. She had also happily learned not to run headlong into trees. More than that, Noreen wrote: 'What you did for her when she broke her neck was an act of heroism that we still find hard to believe – it seems like a miracle every time we look at her.'

I do not consider myself a hero, but I still believe in my own personal hero, Vetman, and in doing our best for all of the animals. Noreen told me that my stethoscope, which I'd given Lev that day we discussed bullying, was one of her son's most treasured possessions, because I had shown him that 'if you have a passion, it gives your life meaning'. 'Most of all,' she added, 'you showed him that you should never give up, that there is always hope, and that the seemingly impossible can actually be achieved if you can push yourself almost beyond your limits.'

Lev was getting along well and changed schools to one where he wasn't bullied, she added. 'He likes science and design technology best … so you never know, he might follow in your footsteps one day!' Noreen has since sent me a picture of Lev and Willow sitting contentedly in their garden, Lev with my stethoscope around his neck and with a big beaming grin on his face.

'The seemingly impossible can be achieved if you can push yourself almost beyond your limits,' Noreen wrote – and of that I have no doubt. As Larry the farmer once said to me, 'everything is impossible until it happens', and as my mammy and my daddy have taught me, the greatest value is not in what you keep for yourself, but what you give to others; and if you work hard enough and believe enough, any dream can come true. Listening to the animals and to all of the people who have loved them has taken me from a profound feeling of helplessness as a child in Ireland to the brink of potentially doing something really important that might improve and extend quality of life for both animals and humans.

There is nothing particularly special about me or my story. I just worked hard, dreamed big and had the conviction to act on my decisions, for better or for worse. I would say to anyone, the greatest thing standing in the way of your dreams is indecision, listening to people who want to bring you down and a lack of certainty about what you really want in life. I'm crystal clear about what I want to achieve – and have been since I was eleven years old. I still have a long way to go yet, though.

I hope to open my third hospital within which we can create, in real life, Vetman's operating theatre, where he healed the animals with the magic bionic stardust of love, that has since manifested as stem cells, which may allow me to rebuild diseased body parts with the perfect marriage of mechanics and biology, just like in my childhood dreams. I hope to help many more ill and injured animals in my life-time. I hope to inspire future generations of vets and doctors. I hope to establish The Humanimal Trust as a hub for One Medicine globally. I hope to translate the love I see between animals and humans in any single home into the homes of animals the world over, before we destroy all their habitats and perhaps even ourselves in the process. I have many hopes.

Not that long ago, I received two letters that moved me deeply, regarding children who had watched *The Supervet*. The first was from a lady in Germany who was looking after a child refugee from the Syrian conflict, called Miro. In his language, Miro's name means 'peace world', but, in his short life, this small boy had seen first-hand the most brutal of wars and had witnessed his mother being raped and killed. The lady wanted to thank me as she said that Miro had watched the same episodes of *The Supervet* on repeat and, even though he had no idea what I actually said, it was obvious they gave him comfort and hope. That meant more than I can say.

The second letter was addressed to 'Mr The Supervet' from a young boy who had come with his mum from 'The Manchester' to see me at 'The Dogfest'. He couldn't talk to me there because, in his words, I was 'too busy hugging and kissing all of the ladies'. He said that he wanted to thank me for 'fixing all of the Nanimals' and advised that he wanted to give me some money for The Humanimal Trust charity. The envelope in which the letter came contained almost three pounds in coins in a tube, which he had earned washing cars. In conclusion, he articulated the reason why I make *The Supervet* in language far more succinct than I could ever have done. He said:

'because I know that when you look after the
Nanimals, you look after me.'

That star I wished upon when I decided I wanted to be a vet aged ten, lying on my back in that ice-starched field and staring up at the enormity of the universe, has been the guiding light of my entire life. For me, one of the brightest stars in heaven is *you* reading this book right now. You have infinite potential and, if enough stars resonate with the same light, I believe we could together change the world for the better. Thank you for giving me the strength, belief and faith I wished for all those years ago. I am deeply grateful to you for picking up this book, for watching the TV show and for thinking about some of the issues that I have raised. As I said at the outset, when I started making *The Supervet*, I never set out to make a show about science, it was always intended to be a show about love and hope. So, thank you for listening to the animals – who give us both of these blessings in abundance.

EPILOGUE

On my thirteenth birthday, 13 December 1980, I made up a poem while sitting in the dark shed of our farmyard with Pirate. It was for Vetman to give to the world because I hoped that he would live on, long after I am no longer around. Like all of the animals, we are merely passing through, and if I could give you one thing in my lifetime it would be this thought, which I have learned from the animals, to keep you safe and to bring you peace:

For when night's pillow nuzzles back the day
The only light you get to keep – is the love you gave
away

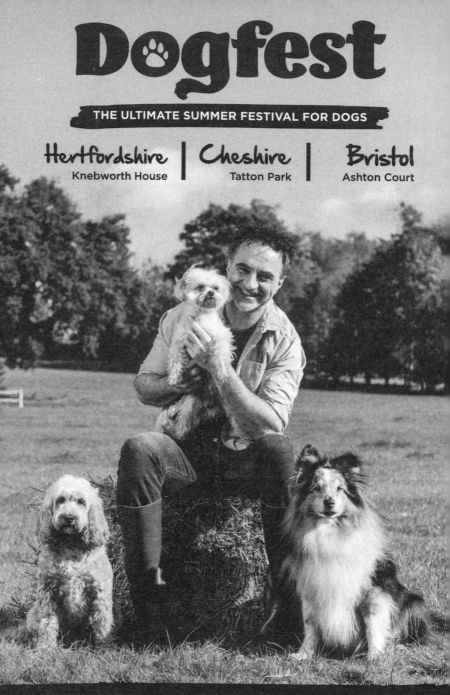